Davi-Ellen Chabner, B.A., M.A.T.

W9-CBT-884

Medical Language
INSTANT
TRANSLATOR

W.B. SAUNDERS COMPANY
A Harcourt Health Sciences Company
Philadelphia   London   New York
St. Louis   Sydney   Toronto

W.B. SAUNDERS COMPANY
A Harcourt Health Sciences Company

The Curtis Center
Independence Square West
Philadelphia, Pennsylvania 19106

Library of Congress Cataloging-in-Publication Data

Chabner, Davi-Ellen.

Medical language instant translator / Davi-Ellen Chabner.

p. ; cm.

Includes index.

ISBN 0–7216–8582–X

1. Medicine—Terminology. 2. Medical sciences—Terminology. I. Title.
[DNLM: 1. Terminology. W 15 C427ma 2001]

R123.C433 2001 610′.1′4–dc21

00-055720

MEDICAL LANGUAGE INSTANT
TRANSLATOR   ISBN 0–7216–8582–X

Printed in the United States of America.

Last digit is the print number:
9   8   7   6   5   4   3   2

WELCOME

This *Medical Language Instant Translator* will provide quick access to useful, medically related information for both laypersons and students entering the health-related professions. Today we are increasingly exposed to medical terminology, whether it be at the doctor's office, on the Internet, or in the media. Being able to analyze and understand these terms allows us to participate in important issues affecting our society as well as to make better decisions about our own health.

Using this handy pocket-size book, you will be able to:

- Decipher complicated medical terms by recognizing and finding the meanings of individual word parts;
- Access information on medical abbreviations, symbols, acronyms, and professional designations;
- Understand the definitions of commonly used diagnostic tests and procedures;
- Identify the top 100 principal medical diagnoses and their associated procedures (also, because this information contains many medical terms, you will get practice analyzing and understanding these terms);
- Identify the top 100 prescription drugs and their uses;
- Interpret the significance of common blood tests;
- Visualize the location of many organs and body structures with full-color illustrations.

Although this *Instant Translator* dovetails with information in both my books, *The Language of Medi-*

cine and *Medical Terminology: A Short Course,* all students of the medical language can benefit from it. Please let me know how the *Instant Translator* works for you and have fun using it!

DAVI-ELLEN CHABNER

CONTENTS

BODY SYSTEMS ILLUSTRATIONS

PART I

THE LANGUAGE OF MEDICINE

How To Analyze
Medical Terms*

Studying medical terminology is very similar to learning a new language. The words at first sound strange and complicated, although they may stand for commonly known English terms. The terms **otalgia**, meaning ear ache, and **ophthalmologist**, meaning eye doctor, are examples.

Your first job in learning the language is to understand how to divide words into their component parts. The medical language is logical in that most terms, whether complex or simple, can be broken down into basic parts and then understood. For example, consider the following term:

HEMATOLOGY	HEMAT/O/LOGY
	↓ ↓
	root suffix
	↓
	combining vowel

The **root** is the *foundation of the word*. All medical terms have one or more roots. The root **hemat** means **blood**.

The **suffix** is the *word ending*. All medical terms have a suffix. The suffix -**logy** means **study of**.

The **combining vowel** (usually o) *links the root to the suffix or the root to another root*. A combining vowel has no meaning of its own; it only joins one word part to another.

It is useful to read the meaning of medical terms *starting from the suffix and moving back to the*

* From Chabner DE: The Language of Medicine, 6th ed. Philadelphia, W.B. Saunders, 2001.

beginning of the term. Thus, the term **hematology** means **study of blood.**

Here is another familiar medical term:

ELECTROCARDIOGRAM

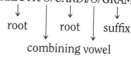

The root **electr** means **electricity.**
The root **cardi** means **heart.**
The suffix **-gram** means **record.**
The entire word means **record of the electricity in the heart.**

Notice that there are two combining vowels in this term. They link the two roots (**electr** and **cardi**) as well as the root (**cardi**) and suffix (**-gram**).

Try another term:

GASTRITIS   GASTR/ITIS
                     ↓   ↓
                   root   suffix

The root **gastr** means **stomach.**
The suffix **-itis** means **inflammation.**

The entire word, reading from the end of the term (suffix) to the beginning, means **inflammation of the stomach.**

Note that the combining vowel, o, is missing in this term. This is because the suffix, -itis, begins with a vowel. The combining vowel is dropped before a suffix that begins with a vowel. It is retained, however, between two roots, even if the second root begins with a vowel. Consider the following term:

GASTROENTEROLOGY

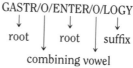

The root **gastr** means **stomach**.
The root **enter** means **intestines**.
The suffix **-logy** means **study of**.
The entire term means **study of the stomach and intestines**.

Notice that the combining vowel is used between **gastr** and **enter**, even though the second root, **enter**, begins with a vowel. When a term contains two or more roots related to parts of the body, often anatomical position determines which root goes before the other. For example, the stomach receives food first, before the small intestine, thus, **gastroenteritis**, not enterogastritis.

In summary, remember three general rules:
1. Read the meaning of medical terms from the suffix back to the beginning of the term and across.
2. Drop the combining vowel (usually o) before a suffix beginning with a vowel: **gastritis** *not* gastroitis.
3. Keep the combining vowel between two roots: **gastroenterology** *not* gastrenterology.

In addition to the root, suffix, and combining vowel, there are two other word parts commonly found in medical terms. These are the **combining form** and **prefix**. The combining form is simply the root plus the combining vowel. For example, you are already familiar with the following combining forms and their meanings:

HEMAT/O   means   **blood**

root + combining vowel = COMBINING FORM

GASTR/O   means   **stomach**

root + combining vowel = COMBINING FORM

CARDI/O   means   **heart**

root + combining vowel = COMBINING FORM

Combining forms can be used with many different suffixes, so it is useful to know the meaning of a combining form to decipher the meaning of a term.

The **prefix** is a small part that is attached to the *beginning of a term*. Not all medical terms contain prefixes, but the prefix can have an important influence on meaning. Consider the following examples:

SUB/GASTR/IC   means   pertaining to under the stomach

prefix   root   suffix
(under) (stomach) (pertaining to)

EPI/GASTR/IC   means   pertaining to above the stomach

prefix   root   suffix
(above) (stomach) (pertaining to)

In summary, the important elements of medical terms are:
1. **Root:** foundation of the term
2. **Suffix:** word ending
3. **Prefix:** word beginning
4. **Combining vowel:** vowel (usually o) that links the root to the suffix or the root to another root
5. **Combining form:** combination of the root and the combining vowel

Glossary of Word Parts Used in Medical Terminology*

Medical Word Parts—English

Combining Form, Suffix, or Prefix	Meaning
a-, an-	no; not; without
ab-	away from
abdomin/o	abdomen
-ac	pertaining to
acanth/o	spiny; thorny
acetabul/o	acetabulum (hip socket)
acous/o	hearing
acr/o	extremities; top; extreme point
acromi/o	acromion (extension of shoulder bone)
actin/o	light
acu/o	sharp; severe; sudden
-acusis	hearing
ad-	toward
aden/o	gland
adenoid/o	adenoids
adip/o	fat
adren/o	adrenal gland
adrenal/o	adrenal gland
aer/o	air
af-	toward
agglutin/o	clumping; sticking together

Chart continued on following page

From Chabner DE: The Language of Medicine, 6th ed. Philadelphia, W.B. Saunders, 2001.

Medical Word Parts—English *Continued*

Combining Form, Suffix, or Prefix	Meaning
-agon	to assemble, gather
agora-	marketplace
-agra	excessive pain
-al	pertaining to
alb/o	white
albin/o	white
albumin/o	albumin (protein)
alges/o	sensitivity to pain
-algesia	sensitivity to pain
-algia	pain
all/o	other
alveol/o	alveolus; air sac; small sac
ambly/o	dim; dull
-amine	nitrogen compound
amni/o	amnion (sac surrounding the embryo)
amyl/o	starch
an/o	anus
-an	pertaining to
ana-	up; apart; backward
andr/o	male
aneurysm/o	aneurysm (widened blood vessel)
angi/o	vessel (blood)
anis/o	unequal
ankyl/o	crooked; bent; stiff
ante-	before; forward
anter/o	front
anthrac/o	coal
anti-	against
anxi/o	uneasy; anxious
aort/o	aorta (largest artery)
-apheresis	removal
aphth/o	ulcer
apo-	off, away
aponeur/o	aponeurosis (type of tendon)

Medical Word Parts—English *Continued*

Combining Form, Suffix, or Prefix	Meaning
append/o	appendix
appendic/o	appendix
aque/o	water
-ar	pertaining to
-arche	beginning
arter/o	artery
arteri/o	artery
arteriol/o	arteriole (small artery)
arthr/o	joint
-arthria	articulate (speak distinctly)
articul/o	joint
-ary	pertaining to
asbest/o	asbestos
-ase	enzyme
-asthenia	lack of strength
atel/o	incomplete
ather/o	plaque (fatty substance)
-ation	process; condition
atri/o	atrium (upper heart chamber)
audi/o	hearing
audit/o	hearing
aur/o	ear
auricul/o	ear
auto-	self, own
axill/o	armpit
azot/o	urea; nitrogen
bacill/o	bacilli (bacteria)
bacteri/o	bacteria
balan/o	glans penis
bar/o	pressure; weight
bartholin/o	Bartholin glands
bas/o	base; opposite of acid

Chart continued on following page

Medical Word Parts—English *Continued*

Combining Form, Suffix, or Prefix	Meaning
bi-	two
bi/o	life
bil/i	bile; gall
bilirubin/o	bilirubin
-blast	embryonic; immature
blephar/o	eyelid
bol/o	cast; throw
brachi/o	arm
brachy-	short
brady-	slow
bronch/o	bronchial tube
bronchi/o	bronchial tube
bronchiol/o	bronchiole
bucc/o	cheek
bunion/o	bunion
burs/o	bursa (sac of fluid near joints)
byssin/o	cotton dust
cac/o	bad
calc/o	calcium
calcane/o	calcaneus (heel bone)
calci/o	calcium
cali/o	calyx
calic/o	calyx
capillar/o	capillary (tiniest blood vessel)
capn/o	carbon dioxide
-capnia	carbon dioxide
carcin/o	cancerous; cancer
cardi/o	heart
carp/o	wrist bones (carpals)
cata-	down
caud/o	tail; lower part of body
caus/o	burn; burning
cauter/o	heat; burn

Medical Word Parts—English *Continued*

Combining Form, Suffix, or Prefix	Meaning
cec/o	cecum (first part of the colon)
-cele	hernia
celi/o	belly; abdomen
-centesis	surgical puncture to remove fluid
cephal/o	head
cerebell/o	cerebellum (posterior part of the brain)
cerebr/o	cerebrum (largest part of the brain)
cerumin/o	cerumen
cervic/o	neck; cervix (neck of uterus)
-chalasia	relaxation
-chalasis	relaxation
cheil/o	lip
chem/o	drug; chemical
-chezia	defecation; elimination of wastes
chir/o	hand
chlor/o	green
chlorhydr/o	hydrochloric acid
chol/e	bile; gall
cholangi/o	bile vessel
cholecyst/o	gallbladder
choledoch/o	common bile duct
cholesterol/o	cholesterol
chondr/o	cartilage
chore/o	dance
chori/o	chorion (outermost membrane of the fetus)
chorion/o	chorion
choroid/o	choroid layer of eye
chrom/o	color
chron/o	time
chym/o	to pour
cib/o	meal
-cide	killing

Chart continued on following page

Medical Word Parts—English *Continued*

Combining Form, Suffix, or Prefix	Meaning
-cidal	pertaining to killing
cine/o	movement
cirrh/o	orange-yellow
cis/o	to cut
-clasis	to break
-clast	to break
claustr/o	enclosed space
clavicul/o	clavicle (collar bone)
-clysis	irrigation; washing
coagul/o	coagulation (clotting)
-coccus (-cocci, pl.)	berry-shaped bacterium
coccyg/o	coccyx (tailbone)
col/o	colon (large intestine)
coll/a	glue
colon/o	colon (large intestine)
colp/o	vagina
comat/o	deep sleep
comi/o	to care for
con-	together, with
coni/o	dust
conjunctiv/o	conjunctiva (lines the eyelids)
-constriction	narrowing
contra-	against; opposite
cor/o	pupil
core/o	pupil
corne/o	cornea
coron/o	heart
corpor/o	body
cortic/o	cortex, outer region
cost/o	rib
crani/o	skull
cras/o	mixture; temperament
crin/o	secrete
-crine	secrete; separate

Medical Word Parts—English *Continued*

Combining Form, Suffix, or Prefix	Meaning
-crit	to separate
cry/o	cold
crypt/o	hidden
culd/o	cul-de-sac
-cusis	hearing
cutane/o	skin
cyan/o	blue
cycl/o	ciliary body of eye; cycle; circle
-cyesis	pregnancy
cyst/o	urinary bladder; cyst; sac of fluid
cyt/o	cell
-cyte	cell
-cytosis	condition of cells; slight increase in numbers
dacry/o	tear
dacryoaden/o	tear gland
dacryocyst/o	tear sac; lacrimal sac
dactyl/o	fingers; toes
de-	lack of; down; less; removal of
dem/o	people
dent/i	tooth
derm/o	skin
-derma	skin
dermat/o	skin
desicc/o	drying
-desis	to bind, tie together
dia-	complete; through
diaphor/o	sweat
-dilation	widening; stretching; expanding
dipl/o	double
dips/o	thirst
dist/o	far; distant

Chart continued on following page

Medical Word Parts—English *Continued*

Combining Form, Suffix, or Prefix	Meaning
dors/o	back (of body)
dorsi-	back
-dote	to give
-drome	to run
duct/o	to lead, carry
duoden/o	duodenum
dur/o	dura mater
-dynia	pain
dys-	bad; painful; difficult; abnormal
-eal	pertaining to
ec-	out; outside
echo-	reflected sound
-ectasia	stretching; dilation; expansion
-ectasis	stretching; dilation; expansion
ecto-	out; outside
-ectomy	removal; excision; resection
-edema	swelling
-elasma	flat plate
electr/o	electricity
em-	in
-ema	condition
-emesis	vomiting
-emia	blood condition
-emic	pertaining to blood condition
emmetr/o	in due measure
en-	in; within
encephal/o	brain
endo-	in; within
enter/o	intestines (usually small intestine)
eosin/o	rosy; dawn-colored
epi-	above; upon; on
epididym/o	epididymis
epiglott/o	epiglottis

Medical Word Parts—English *Continued*

Combining Form, Suffix, or Prefix	Meaning
episi/o	vulva (external female genitalia)
epitheli/o	skin; epithelium
equin/o	horse
-er	one who
erg/o	work
erythem/o	flushed; redness
erythr/o	red
-esis	condition
eso-	inward
esophag/o	esophagus
esthes/o	nervous sensation (feeling)
esthesi/o	nervous sensation
-esthesia	nervous sensation
estr/o	female
ethm/o	sieve
eti/o	cause
eu-	good; normal
-eurysm	widening
ex-	out; away from
exanthemat/o	rash
exo-	out; away from
extra-	outside
faci/o	face
fasci/o	fascia (membrane supporting muscles)
femor/o	femur (thigh bone)
-ferent	to carry
fibr/o	fiber
fibros/o	fibrous connective tissue
fibul/o	fibula
-fication	process of making
-fida	split

Chart continued on following page

Medical Word Parts—English *Continued*

Combining Form, Suffix, or Prefix	Meaning
flex/o	to bend
fluor/o	luminous
follicul/o	follicle; small sac
-form	resembling; in the shape of
fung/i	fungus; mushroom
furc/o	forking; branching
-fusion	to pour
galact/o	milk
ganglion/o	ganglion; collection of nerve cell bodies
gastr/o	stomach
-gen	producing; forming
-genesis	producing; forming
-genic	produced by or in
ger/o	old age
gest/o	pregnancy
gester/o	pregnancy
gingiv/o	gum
glauc/o	gray
gli/o	glue; neuroglial tissue (supportive tissue of nervous system)
-globin	protein
-globulin	protein
glomerul/o	glomerulus
gloss/o	tongue
gluc/o	glucose; sugar
glyc/o	glucose; sugar
glycogen/o	glycogen; animal starch
glycos/o	glucose; sugar
gnos/o	knowledge
gon/o	seed
gonad/o	sex glands
goni/o	angle

Medical Word Parts—English *Continued*

Combining Form, Suffix, or Prefix	Meaning
-grade	to go
-gram	record
granul/o	granule(s)
-graph	instrument for recording
-graphy	process of recording
gravid/o	pregnancy
-gravida	pregnant woman
gynec/o	woman; female
hallucin/o	hallucination
hem/o	blood
hemat/o	blood
hemi-	half
hemoglobin/o	hemoglobin
hepat/o	liver
herni/o	hernia
-hexia	habit
hidr/o	sweat
hist/o	tissue
histi/o	tissue
home/o	sameness; unchanging; constant
hormon/o	hormone
humer/o	humerus (upper arm bone)
hydr/o	water
hyper-	above; excessive
hypn/o	sleep
hypo-	deficient; below; under
hypophys/o	pituitary gland
hyster/o	uterus; womb
-ia	condition
-iac	pertaining to

Chart continued on following page

Medical Word Parts—English *Continued*

Combining Form, Suffix, or Prefix	Meaning
-iasis	abnormal condition
iatr/o	physician; treatment
-ic	pertaining to
-ical	pertaining to
ichthy/o	dry; scaly
-icle	small
idi/o	unknown; individual; distinct
ile/o	ileum (part of small intestine)
ili/o	ilium (part of hip bone)
immun/o	immune; protection; safe
in-	in; into; not
-in, -ine	a substance
-ine	pertaining to
infra-	below; inferior to; beneath
inguin/o	groin
inter-	between
intra-	within; into
iod/o	iodine
ion/o	ion; to wander
-ion	process
-ior	pertaining to
ipsi-	same
ir-	in
ir/o	iris (colored portion of eye)
irid/o	iris (colored portion of eye)
is/o	same; equal
isch/o	to hold back; back
ischi/o	ischium (part of hip bone)
-ism	process; condition
-ist	specialist
-itis	inflammation
-ium	structure; tissue
jaund/o	yellow
jejun/o	jejunum

Medical Word Parts—English *Continued*

Combining Form, Suffix, or Prefix	Meaning
kal/i	potassium
kary/o	nucleus
kerat/o	horny, hard; cornea
kern-	nucleus (collection of nerve cells in the brain)
ket/o	ketones; acetones
keton/o	ketones; acetones
kines/o	movement
kinesi/o	movement
-kinesia	movement
-kinesis	movement
klept/o	to steal
kyph/o	humpback
labi/o	lip
lacrim/o	tear; tear duct; lacrimal duct
lact/o	milk
lamin/o	lamina (part of vertebral arch)
lapar/o	abdominal wall; abdomen
-lapse	to slide, fall, sag
laryng/o	larynx (voice box)
later/o	side
leiomy/o	smooth (visceral) muscle
-lemma	sheath, covering
-lepsy	seizure
lept/o	thin, slender
-leptic	to seize, take hold of
leth/o	death
leuk/o	white
lute/o	yellow
lex/o	word; phrase
-lexia	word; phrase
ligament/o	ligament

Chart continued on following page

Medical Word Parts—English *Continued*

Combining Form, Suffix, or Prefix	Meaning
lingu/o	tongue
lip/o	fat; lipid
-listhesis	slipping
lith/o	stone; calculus
-lithiasis	condition of stones
-lithotomy	incision (for removal) of a stone
lob/o	lobe
log/o	study of
-logy	study of
lord/o	curve; swayback
-lucent	to shine
lumb/o	lower back; loin
lute/o	yellow
lux/o	to slide
lymph/o	lymph
lymphaden/o	lymph gland (node)
lymphangi/o	lymph vessel
-lysis	breakdown; separation; destruction; loosening
-lytic	to reduce, destroy
macro-	large
mal-	bad
-malacia	softening
malleol/o	malleolus
mamm/o	breast
mandibul/o	mandible (lower jaw bone)
-mania	obsessive preoccupation
mast/o	breast
mastoid/o	mastoid process (behind the ear)
maxill/o	maxilla (upper jaw bone)
meat/o	meatus (opening)
medi/o	middle
mediastin/o	mediastinum

Medical Word Parts—English *Continued*

Combining Form, Suffix, or Prefix	Meaning
medull/o	medulla (inner section); middle; soft, marrow
mega-	large
-megaly	enlargement
melan/o	black
men/o	menses; menstruation
mening/o	meninges (membranes covering the spinal cord and brain)
meningi/o	meninges
ment/o	mind; chin
meso-	middle
meta-	change; beyond
metacarp/o	metacarpals (hand bones)
metatars/o	metatarsals (foot bones)
-meter	measure
metr/o	uterus (womb); measure
metri/o	uterus (womb)
mi/o	smaller; less
micro-	small
-mimetic	mimic; copy
-mission	to send
mon/o	one; single
morph/o	shape; form
mort/o	death
-mortem	death
-motor	movement
muc/o	mucus
mucos/o	mucous membrane (mucosa)
multi-	many
mut/a	genetic change
mutagen/o	causing genetic change
my/o	muscle
myc/o	fungus
mydr/o	wide

Chart continued on following page

Medical Word Parts—English *Continued*

Combining Form, Suffix, or Prefix	Meaning
myel/o	spinal cord; bone marrow
myocardi/o	myocardium (heart muscle)
myom/o	muscle tumor
myos/o	muscle
myring/o	tympanic membrane (eardrum)
myx/o	mucus
narc/o	numbness; stupor; sleep
nas/o	nose
nat/i	birth
natr/o	sodium
necr/o	death
nect/o	to bind, tie, connect
neo-	new
nephr/o	kidney
neur/o	nerve
neutr/o	neither; neutral
nid/o	nest
noct/i	night
norm/o	rule; order
nos/o	disease
nucle/o	nucleus
nulli-	none
nyct/o	night
obstetr/o	midwife
ocul/o	eye
odont/o	tooth
odyn/o	pain
-oid	resembling
-ole	little; small
olecran/o	olecranon (elbow)
olig/o	scanty

Medical Word Parts—English *Continued*

Combining Form, Suffix, or Prefix	Meaning
om/o	shoulder
-oma	tumor; mass; fluid collection
omphal/o	umbilicus (navel)
onc/o	tumor
-one	hormone
onych/o	nail (of fingers or toes)
o/o	egg
oophor/o	ovary
-opaque	obscure
ophthalm/o	eye
-opia	vision
-opsia	vision
-opsy	view of
opt/o	eye; vision
optic/o	eye; vision
-or	one who
or/o	mouth
orch/o	testis
orchi/o	testis
orchid/o	testis
-orexia	appetite
orth/o	straight
-ose	full of; pertaining to; sugar
-osis	condition, usually abnormal
-osmia	smell
ossicul/o	ossicle (small bone)
oste/o	bone
-ostosis	condition of bone
ot/o	ear
-otia	ear condition
-ous	pertaining to
ov/o	egg
ovari/o	ovary
ovul/o	egg

Chart continued on following page

Medical Word Parts—English *Continued*

Combining Form, Suffix, or Prefix	Meaning
ox/o	oxygen
-oxia	oxygen
oxy-	swift; sharp; acid
oxysm/o	sudden
pachy-	heavy; thick
palat/o	palate (roof of the mouth)
palpebr/o	eyelid
pan-	all
pancreat/o	pancreas
papill/o	nipple-like; optic disc (disk)
par-	other than; abnormal
para-	near; beside; abnormal; apart from; along the side of
-para	to bear, bring forth (live births)
-parous	to bear, bring forth
parathyroid/o	parathyroid glands
-paresis	slight paralysis
-pareunia	sexual intercourse
-partum	birth; labor
patell/a	patella (kneecap)
patell/o	patella
path/o	disease
-pathy	disease; emotion
pector/o	chest
ped/o	child; foot
pelv/i	pelvic bone; hip
pend/o	to hang
-penia	deficiency
-pepsia	digestion
per-	through
peri-	surrounding
perine/o	perineum
peritone/o	peritoneum

Medical Word Parts—English *Continued*

Combining Form, Suffix, or Prefix	Meaning
perone/o	fibula
-pexy	fixation; to put in place
phac/o	lens of eye
phag/o	eat; swallow
-phage	eat; swallow
-phagia	eating; swallowing
phak/o	lens of eye
phalang/o	phalanges (fingers and toes)
phall/o	penis
pharmac/o	drug
pharmaceut/o	drug
pharyng/o	throat (pharynx)
phas/o	speech
-phasia	speech
phe/o	dusky; dark
-pheresis	removal
phil/o	like; love; attraction to
-phil	attraction for
-philia	attraction for
phim/o	muzzle
phleb/o	vein
phob/o	fear
-phobia	fear
phon/o	voice; sound
-phonia	voice; sound
-phor/o	to bear
-phoresis	carrying; transmission
-phoria	to bear, carry; feeling (mental state)
phot/o	light
phren/o	diaphragm; mind
-phthisis	wasting away
-phylaxis	protection
physi/o	nature; function
-physis	to grow

Chart continued on following page

Medical Word Parts—English *Continued*

Combining Form, Suffix, or Prefix	Meaning
phyt/o	plant
-phyte	plant
pil/o	hair
pineal/o	pineal gland
pituitar/o	pituitary gland
-plakia	plaque
plant/o	sole of the foot
plas/o	development; formation
-plasia	development; formation; growth
-plasm	formation
-plastic	pertaining to formation
-plasty	surgical repair
ple/o	more; many
-plegia	paralysis; palsy
-plegic	paralysis; palsy
pleur/o	pleura
plex/o	plexus; network (of nerves)
-pnea	breathing
pneum/o	lung; air; gas
pneumon/o	lung; air; gas
pod/o	foot
-poiesis	formation
-poietin	substance that forms
poikil/o	varied; irregular
pol/o	extreme
polio-	gray matter (of brain or spinal cord)
poly-	many; much
polyp/o	polyp; small growth
pont/o	pons (a part of the brain)
-porosis	condition of pores (spaces)
post-	after; behind
poster/o	back (of body); behind
-prandial	meal
-praxia	action

Medical Word Parts—English *Continued*

Combining Form, Suffix, or Prefix	Meaning
pre-	before; in front of
presby/o	old age
primi-	first
pro-	before; forward
proct/o	anus and rectum
pros-	before; forward
prostat/o	prostate gland
prot/o	first
prote/o	protein
proxim/o	near
prurit/o	itching
pseudo-	false
psych/o	mind
-ptosis	droop; sag; prolapse; fall
-ptysis	spitting
pub/o	pubis (anterior part of hip bone)
pulmon/o	lung
pupill/o	pupil (dark center of the eye)
purul/o	pus
py/o	pus
pyel/o	renal pelvis
pylor/o	pylorus; pyloric sphincter
pyr/o	fever; fire
pyret/o	fever
pyrex/o	fever
quadri-	four
rachi/o	spinal column; vertebrae
radi/o	x-rays; radioactivity; radius (lateral lower arm bone)
radicul/o	nerve root

Chart continued on following page

Medical Word Parts—English *Continued*

Combining Form, Suffix, or Prefix	Meaning
re-	back; again; backward
rect/o	rectum
ren/o	kidney
reticul/o	network
retin/o	retina
retro-	behind; back; backward
rhabdomy/o	striated (skeletal) muscle
rheumat/o	watery flow (in joints)
rhin/o	nose
roentgen/o	x-rays
-rrhage	bursting forth of blood
-rrhagia	bursting forth of blood
-rrhaphy	suture
-rrhea	flow; discharge
-rrhexis	rupture
rrhythm/o	rhythm
sacr/o	sacrum
salping/o	fallopian tube; auditory (eustachian) tube
-salpinx	fallopian tube; oviduct
sarc/o	flesh (connective tissue)
scapul/o	scapula; shoulder blade
-schisis	to split
schiz/o	split
scint/i	spark
scirrh/o	hard
scler/o	sclera (white of the eye)
-sclerosis	hardening
scoli/o	crooked; bent
-scope	instrument for visual examination
-scopy	visual examination
scot/o	darkness
seb/o	sebum

Medical Word Parts—English *Continued*

Combining Form, Suffix, or Prefix	Meaning
sebace/o	sebum
sect/o	to cut
semi-	half
semin/i	semen; seed
seps/o	infection
sial/o	saliva
sialaden/o	salivary gland
sider/o	iron
sigmoid/o	sigmoid colon
silic/o	glass
sinus/o	sinus
-sis	state of; condition
-sol	solution
somat/o	body
-some	body
somn/o	sleep
-somnia	sleep
son/o	sound
-spadia	to tear, cut
-spasm	sudden contraction of muscles
sperm/o	spermatozoa; sperm cells
spermat/o	spermatozoa; sperm cells
sphen/o	wedge; sphenoid bone
spher/o	globe-shaped; round
sphygm/o	pulse
-sphyxia	pulse
spin/o	spine (backbone)
spir/o	to breathe
splen/o	spleen
spondyl/o	vertebra (backbone)
squam/o	scale
-stalsis	contraction
staped/o	stapes (middle ear bone)
staphyl/o	clusters; uvula

Chart continued on following page

Medical Word Parts—English *Continued*

Combining Form, Suffix, or Prefix	Meaning
-stasis	stop; control; place
-static	pertaining to stopping; controlling
steat/o	fat, sebum
-stenosis	tightening; stricture
ster/o	solid structure; steroid
stere/o	solid; three-dimensional
stern/o	sternum (breastbone)
steth/o	chest
-sthenia	strength
-stitial	to set; pertaining to standing or positioned
stomat/o	mouth
-stomy	new opening (to form a mouth)
strept/o	twisted chains
styl/o	pole or stake
sub-	under; below
submaxill/o	mandible (lower jaw bone)
-suppression	to stop
supra-	above, upper
sym-	together; with
syn-	together; with
syncop/o	to cut off, cut short
syndesm/o	ligament
synov/o	synovia; synovial membrane; sheath around a tendon
syring/o	tube
tachy-	fast
tars/o	tarsus; hindfoot or ankle (7 bones between the foot and the leg)
tax/o	order; coordination
tel/o	complete
tele/o	distant

Medical Word Parts—English *Continued*

Combining Form, Suffix, or Prefix	Meaning
ten/o	tendon
tendin/o	tendon
-tension	pressure
terat/o	monster; malformed fetus
test/o	testis (testicle)
tetra-	four
thalam/o	thalamus
thalass/o	sea
the/o	put; place
thec/o	sheath
thel/o	nipple
therapeut/o	treatment
-therapy	treatment
therm/o	heat
thorac/o	chest
-thorax	chest; pleural cavity
thromb/o	clot
thym/o	thymus gland
-thymia	mind (condition of)
-thymic	pertaining to mind
thyr/o	thyroid gland; shield
thyroid/o	thyroid gland
tibi/o	tibia (shin bone)
-tic	pertaining to
toc/o	labor; birth
-tocia	labor; birth (condition of)
-tocin	labor; birth (a substance for)
tom/o	to cut
-tome	instrument to cut
-tomy	process of cutting
ton/o	tension
tone/o	to stretch
tonsill/o	tonsil
top/o	place; position; location

Chart continued on following page

Medical Word Parts—English *Continued*

Combining Form, Suffix, or Prefix	Meaning
tox/o	poison
toxic/o	poison
trache/o	trachea (windpipe)
trans-	across; through
-tresia	opening
tri-	three
trich/o	hair
trigon/o	trigone (area within the bladder)
-tripsy	to crush
troph/o	nourishment; development
-trophy	nourishment; development
-tropia	to turn
-tropic	turning
-tropin	stimulate; act on
tympan/o	tympanic membrane (eardrum); middle ear
-type	classification; picture
-ule	little; small
uln/o	ulna (medial lower arm bone)
ultra-	beyond; excess
-um	structure; tissue; thing
umbilic/o	umbilicus (navel)
ungu/o	nail
uni-	one
ur/o	urine; urinary tract
ureter/o	ureter
urethr/o	urethra
-uria	urination; condition of urine
urin/o	urine
-us	structure; thing
uter/o	uterus (womb)
uve/o	uvea, vascular layer of eye (iris, choroid, ciliary body)
uvul/o	uvula

Medical Word Parts—English *Continued*

Combining Form, Suffix, or Prefix	Meaning
vag/o	vagus nerve
vagin/o	vagina
valv/o	valve
valvul/o	valve
varic/o	varicose veins
vas/o	vessel; duct; vas deferens
vascul/o	vessel (blood)
ven/o	vein
ventr/o	belly side of body
ventricul/o	ventricle (of heart or brain)
venul/o	venule (small vein)
-verse	to turn
-version	to turn
vertebr/o	vertebra (backbone)
vesic/o	urinary bladder
vesicul/o	seminal vesicle
vestibul/o	vestibule of the inner ear
viscer/o	internal organs
vit/o	life
vitr/o	vitreous body (of the eye)
vitre/o	glass
viv/o	life
vol/o	to roll
vulv/o	vulva (female external genitalia)
xanth/o	yellow
xen/o	stranger
xer/o	dry
xiph/o	sword
-y	condition; process
zo/o	animal life

English—Medical Word Parts

Meaning	Combining Form, Prefix, or Suffix
abdomen	abdomin/o (use with -al, -centesis)
	celi/o (use with -ac)
	lapar/o (use with -scope, -scopy, -tomy)
abdominal wall	lapar/o
abnormal	dys-
	par-
	para-
abnormal condition	-iasis
	-osis
above	epi-
	hyper-
	supra-
acetabulum	acetabul/o
acetones	ket/o
	keton/o
acid	oxy-
acromion	acromi/o
across	trans-
action	-praxia
act on	-tropin
adrenal glands	adren/o
	adrenal/o
after	post-
again	re-
against	anti-
	contra-
air	aer/o
	pneum/o
	pneumon/o
air sac	alveol/o
albumin	albumin/o
all	pan-
along the side of	para-

English—Medical Word Parts *Continued*

Meaning	Combining Form, Prefix, or Suffix
alveolus	alveol/o
amnion	amni/o
aneurysm	aneurysm/o
angle	goni/o
animal life	zo/o
animal starch	glycogen/o
ankle	tars/o
anus	an/o
anus and rectum	proct/o
anxiety	anxi/o
apart	ana-
apart from	para-
appendix	append/o (use with -ectomy)
	appendic/o (use with -itis)
appetite	-orexia
arm	brachi/o
arm bone, lower, lateral	radi/o
arm bone, lower, medial	uln/o
arm bone, upper	humer/o
armpit	axill/o
arteriole	arteriol/o
artery	arter/o
	arteri/o
articulate (speak distinctly)	-arthria
asbestos	asbest/o
assemble	-agon
atrium	atri/o
attraction for	-phil
	-philia
attraction to	phil/o
auditory tube	salping/o

Chart continued on following page

English—Medical Word Parts *Continued*

Meaning	Combining Form, Prefix, or Suffix
away from	ab-
	apo-
	ex-
	exo-
back	re-
	retro-
back, lower	lumb/o
back portion of body	dorsi-
	dors/o
	poster/o
backbone	spin/o (use with -al)
	spondyl/o (use with -itis, -listhesis, -osis, -pathy)
	vertebr/o (use with -al)
backward	ana-
	retro-
bacteria	bacteri/o
bacterium (berry-shaped)	-coccus (-cocci, pl.)
bacilli (rod-shaped bacteria)	bacill/o
bad	cac/o
	dys-
	mal-
barrier	claustr/o
base (not acidic)	bas/o
bear (to)	-para
	-parous
	-phoria
	phor/o
before	ante-
	pre-
	pro-
	pros-

English—**Medical Word Parts** *Continued*

Meaning	Combining Form, Prefix, or Suffix
beginning	-arche
behind	post-
	poster/o
	retro-
belly	celi/o
belly side of body	ventr/o
below, beneath	hypo-
	infra-
	sub-
bend (to)	flex/o
bent	ankyl/o
	scoli/o
beside	para-
between	inter-
beyond	hyper-
	meta-
	ultra-
bile	bil/i
	chol/e
bile vessel	cholangi/o
bilirubin	bilirubin/o
bind	-desis
	nect/o
birth	nat/i
	-partum
	toc/o
	-tocia
birth (substance for)	-tocin
births (live)	-para
black	anthrac/o, melan/o
bladder (urinary)	cyst/o (use with -ic, -itis, -cele, -gram, -scopy, -stomy, -tomy)
	vesic/o (use with -al)

Chart continued on following page

English—Medical Word Parts *Continued*

Meaning	Combining Form, Prefix, or Suffix
blood	hem/o (use with -dialysis, -globin, -lysis, -philia, -ptysis, -rrhage, -stasis, -stat) hemat/o (use with -crit, -emesis, -logist, -logy, -oma, -poiesis, -uria)
blood condition	-emia
	-emic
blood vessel	angi/o (use with -ectomy, -genesis, -gram, -graphy, -oma, -plasty, -spasm) vas/o (use with -constriction, -dilation, -motor) vascul/o (use with -ar, -itis)
blue	cyan/o
body	corpor/o somat/o -some
bone	oste/o
bone condition	-ostosis
bone marrow	myel/o
brain	encephal/o cerebr/o
branching	furc/o
break	-clasis -clast
breakdown	-lysis
breast	mamm/o (use with -ary, -gram, -graphy, -plasty) mast/o (use with -algia, -dynia, -ectomy, -itis)

English—Medical Word Parts *Continued*

Meaning	Combining Form, Prefix, or Suffix
breastbone	stern/o
breathe	spir/o
breathing	-pnea
bring forth	-para
	-parous
bronchial tube	bronch/o
(bronchus)	bronchi/o
bronchiole	bronchiol/o
bunion	bunion/o
burn	caus/o
	cauter/o
bursa	burs/o
bursting forth of blood	-rrhage
	-rrhagia
calcaneus	calcane/o
calcium	calc/o
	calci/o
calculus	lith/o
calyx	cali/o
	calic/o
cancerous	carcin/o
capillary	capillar/o
carbon dioxide	capn/o
	-capnia
care for (to)	comi/o
carry	duct/o
	-ferent
	-phoria
carrying	-phoresis
cartilage	chondr/o
cast; throw	bol/o
cause	eti/o

Chart continued on following page

English—Medical Word Parts *Continued*

Meaning	Combining Form, Prefix, or Suffix
cecum	cec/o
cell	cyt/o
	-cyte
cells, condition of	-cytosis
cerebellum	cerebell/o
cerebrum	cerebr/o
cerumen	cerumin/o
cervix	cervic/o
change	meta-
cheek	bucc/o
chemical	chem/o
chest	pector/o
	steth/o
	thorac/o
	-thorax
child	ped/o
chin	ment/o
cholesterol	cholesterol/o
chorion	chori/o
	chorion/o
choroid layer (of the eye)	choroid/o
ciliary body (of the eye)	cycl/o
circle or cycle	cycl/o
clavicle (collar bone)	clavicul/o
clot	thromb/o
clumping	agglutin/o
clusters	staphyl/o
coagulation	coagul/o
coal dust	anthrac/o
coccyx	coccyg/o
cold	cry/o
collar bone	clavicul/o
colon	col/o (use with -ectomy, -itis, -pexy, -stomy)
	colon/o (use with -ic, -pathy, -scope, -scopy)

English—Medical Word Parts *Continued*

Meaning	Combining Form, Prefix, or Suffix
color	chrom/o
common bile duct	choledoch/o
complete	dia-
	tel/o
condition	-ation
	-ema
	-esis
	-ia
	-ism
	-sis
	-y
condition, abnormal	-iasis
	-osis
connect	nect/o
connective tissue	sarc/o
constant	home/o
control	-stasis, -stat
contraction	-stalsis
contraction of muscles, sudden	-spasm
coordination	tax/o
copy	-mimetic
cornea (of the eye)	corne/o
	kerat/o
cortex	cortic/o
cotton dust	byssin/o
crooked	ankyl/o
	scoli/o
crush (to)	-tripsy
curve	lord/o
cut	cis/o
	sect/o, -section
	tom/o
cut off	syncop/o
cutting, process of	-tomy

Chart continued on following page

English—Medical Word Parts *Continued*

Meaning	Combining Form, Prefix, or Suffix
cycle	cycl/o
cyst (sac of fluid)	cyst/o
dance	chore/o
dark	phe/o
darkness	scot/o
dawn-colored	eosin/o
death	leth/o
	mort/o, -mortem
	necr/o
defecation	-chezia
deficiency	-penia
deficient	hypo-
destroy	-lytic
destruction	-lysis
development	plas/o
	-plasia
	troph/o
	-trophy
diaphragm	phren/o
difficult	dys-
digestion	-pepsia
dilation	-ectasia
	-ectasis
dim	ambly/o
discharge	-rrhea
disease	nos/o
	path/o
	-pathy
distant	dist/o
	tele/o
distinct	idi/o
double	dipl/o
down	cata-
	de-

English—Medical Word Parts *Continued*

Meaning	Combining Form, Prefix, or Suffix
droop	-ptosis
drug	chem/o
	pharmac/o
	pharmaceut/o
dry	ichthy/o
	xer/o
drying	desicc/o
duct	vas/o
dull	ambly/o
duodenum	duoden/o
dura mater	dur/o
dusky	phe/o
dust	coni/o
ear	aur/o (use with -al, -icle)
	auricul/o (use with -ar)
	ot/o (use with -algia, -ic,
	-itis, -logy, -mycosis,
	-rrhea, -sclerosis, -scope,
	-scopy)
ear (condition of)	-otia
eardrum	myring/o (use with
	-ectomy, -itis, -tomy)
	tympan/o (use with -ic,
	-metry, -plasty)
eat	phag/o
	-phage
eating	-phagia
egg cell	o/o
	ov/o
	ovul/o
elbow	olecran/o
electricity	electr/o
elimination of wastes	-chezia

Chart continued on following page

English—Medical Word Parts *Continued*

Meaning	Combining Form, Prefix, or Suffix
embryonic	-blast
enlargement	-megaly
enzyme	-ase
epididymis	epididym/o
epiglottis	epiglott/o
equal	is/o
esophagus	esophag/o
eustachian tube	salping/o
excess	ultra-
excessive	hyper-
excision	-ectomy
expansion	-ectasia
	-ectasis
extreme	pol/o
extreme point	acr/o
extremities	acr/o
eye	ocul/o (use with -ar, -facial, -motor)
	ophthalm/o (use with -ia, -ic, -logist, -logy, -pathy, -plasty, -plegia, -scope, -scopy)
	opt/o (use with -ic, -metrist)
	optic/o (use with -al, -ian)
eyelid	blephar/o (use with -chalasis, -itis, -plasty, -plegia, -ptosis, -tomy)
	palpebr/o (use with -al)
face	faci/o
fall	-ptosis
fallopian tube	salping/o
	-salpinx

English—Medical Word Parts *Continued*

Meaning	Combining Form, Prefix, or Suffix
false	pseudo-
far	dist/o
fascia	fasci/o
fast	tachy-
fat	adip/o (use with -ose, -osis)
	lip/o (use with -ase, -cyte, -genesis, -oid, -oma)
	steat/o (use with -oma, -rrhea)
fear	phob/o
	-phobia
feeling	esthesi/o
	-phoria
female	estr/o (use with -gen, -genic)
	gynec/o (use with -logist, -logy, -mastia)
femur	femor/o
fever	pyr/o
	pyret/o
	pyrex/o
fiber	fibr/o
fibrous connective tissue	fibros/o
fibula	fibul/o (use with -ar)
	perone/o (use with -al)
finger and toe bones	phalang/o
fingers	dactyl/o
fire	pyr/o
first	prot/o
fixation	-pexy
flat plate	-elasma
flesh	sarc/o

Chart continued on following page

English—Medical Word Parts *Continued*

Meaning	Combining Form, Prefix, or Suffix
flow	-rrhea
fluid collection	-oma
flushed	erythem/o
foot	pod/o
foot bones	metatars/o
forking	furc/o
form	morph/o
formation	plas/o
	-plasia
	-plasm
	-poiesis
forming	-genesis
forward	ante-, pro-, pros-
four	quadri-
front	anter/o
full of	-ose
fungus	fung/i (use with -cide, -oid, -ous, -stasis)
	myc/o (use with -logist, -logy, -osis, -tic)
gall	bil/i (use with -ary)
	chol/e (use with -lithiasis)
gallbladder	cholecyst/o
ganglion	gangli/o
	ganglion/o
gas	pneum/o
	pneumon/o
gather	-agon
genetic change	mut/a
	mutagen/o
give (to)	-dote

English—Medical Word Parts *Continued*

Meaning	Combining Form, Prefix, or Suffix
given (what is)	-dote
gland	aden/o
glans penis	balan/o
glass	silic/o
	vitre/o
globe-shaped	spher/o
glomerulus	glomerul/o
glucose	gluc/o
	glyc/o
	glycos/o
glue	coll/a
	gli/o
glycogen	glycogen/o
go (to)	-grade
good	eu-
granule(s)	granul/o
gray	glauc/o
gray matter	poli/o
green	chlor/o
groin	inguin/o
grow	-physis
growth	-plasia
gum	gingiv/o
habit	-hexia
hair	pil/o
	trich/o
half	hemi-
	semi-
hallucination	hallucin/o
hand	chir/o
hand bones	metacarp/o
hang (to)	pend/o

Chart continued on following page

English—Medical Word Parts *Continued*

Meaning	Combining Form, Prefix, or Suffix
hard	kerat/o
	scirrh/o
hardening	-sclerosis
head	cephal/o
hearing	acous/o
	audi/o
	audit/o
	-acusis
	-cusis
heart	cardi/o (use with -ac, -graphy, -logy, -logist, -megaly, -pathy, -vascular)
	coron/o (use with -ary)
heart muscle	myocardi/o
heat	cauter/o
	therm/o
heavy	pachy-
heel bone	calcane/o
hemoglobin	hemoglobin/o
hernia	-cele
	herni/o
hidden	crypt/o
hip	pelv/i
hold back	isch/o
hormone	hormon/o
	-one
horny	kerat/o
horse	equin/o
humerus	humer/o
humpback	kyph/o
hydrochloric acid	chlorhydr/o
ileum	ile/o
ilium	ili/o

English—Medical Word Parts *Continued*

Meaning	Combining Form, Prefix, or Suffix
immature	-blast
immune	immun/o
in, into	em-
	en-
	endo-
	in-, intra-
	ir-
in due measure	emmetr/o
in front of	pre-
incomplete	atel/o
increase in numbers (blood cells)	-cytosis
individual	idi/o
infection	seps/o
inferior to	infra-
inflammation	-itis
instrument for recording	-graph
instrument for visual examination	-scope
instrument to cut	-tome
internal organs	viscer/o
intestine, large	col/o
intestine, small	enter/o
iodine	iod/o
ion	ion/o
iris	ir/o
	irid/o
iron	sider/o
irregular	poikil/o
irrigation	-clysis
ischium	ischi/o
itching	prurit/o
jaw, lower	mandibul/o
	submaxill/o

Chart continued on following page

English—Medical Word Parts *Continued*

Meaning	Combining Form, Prefix, or Suffix
jaw, upper	maxill/o
joint	arthr/o
	articul/o
ketones	ket/o
	keton/o
kidney	nephr/o (use with -algia, -ectomy, -ic, -itis, -lith, -megaly, -oma, -osis, -pathy, -ptosis, -sclerosis, -stomy, -tomy)
	ren/o (use with -al, -gram, -vascular)
killing	-cidal
	-cide
knowledge	gnos/o
labor	-partum
	toc/o
	-tocia
labor (substance for)	-tocin
lack of	de-
lack of strength	-asthenia
lacrimal duct	dacry/o
	lacrim/o
lacrimal sac	dacryocyst/o
lamina	lamin/o
large	macro-
	mega-
larynx	laryng/o
lead (to)	duct/o
lens of eye	phac/o
	phak/o

English—Medical Word Parts *Continued*

Meaning	Combining Form, Prefix, or Suffix
less	de- mi/o
life	bi/o vit/o viv/o
ligament	ligament/o syndesm/o
like	phil/o
lip	cheil/o labi/o
lipid	lip/o
little	-ole -ule
liver	hepat/o
lobe	lob/o
location	top/o
loin	lumb/o
loosening	-lysis
love	phil/o
luminous	fluor/o
lung	pneum/o (use with -coccus, -coniosis, -thorax) pneumon/o (use with -ectomy, -ia, -ic, -itis, -lysis) pulmon/o (use with -ary)
lymph	lymph/o
lymph gland	lymphaden/o
lymph vessel	lymphangi/o
make (to)	-fication
male	andr/o

Chart continued on following page

English—Medical Word Parts *Continued*

Meaning	Combining Form, Prefix, or Suffix
malformed fetus	terat/o
malleolus	malleol/o
mandible	mandibul/o
	submaxill/o
many	multi-
	ple/o
	poly-
marketplace	agora-
marrow	medull/o
mass	-oma
mastoid process	mastoid/o
maxilla	maxill/o
meal	cib/o
	-prandial
measure	-meter
	metr/o
meatus	meat/o
mediastinum	mediastin/o
medulla oblongata	medull/o
meninges	mening/o
	meningi/o
menstruation; menses	men/o
metacarpals	metacarp/o
metatarsals	metatars/o
middle	medi/o
	medull/o
	meso-
middle ear	tympan/o
midwife	obstetr/o
milk	galact/o
	lact/o
mimic	-mimetic
mind	ment/o
	phren/o
	psych/o
	-thymia
	-thymic

English—Medical Word Parts *Continued*

Meaning	Combining Form, Prefix, or Suffix
mixture	cras/o
monster	terat/o
more	ple/o
mouth	or/o (use with -al)
	stomat/o (use with -itis)
movement	cine/o
	kines/o
	kinesi/o
	-kinesia
	-kinesis
	-motor
much	poly-
mucous membrane	mucos/o
mucus	muc/o
	myx/o
muscle	muscul/o (use with -ar, -skeletal)
	my/o (use with -algia, -ectomy, -oma, -neural, -pathy, -rrhaphy, -therapy)
	myos/o (use with -in, -itis)
muscle, heart	myocardi/o
muscle, smooth (visceral)	leiomy/o
muscle, striated (skeletal)	rhabdomy/o
muscle tumor	myom/o
muzzle	phim/o
nail	onych/o
	ungu/o

Chart continued on following page

English—Medical Word Parts *Continued*

Meaning	Combining Form, Prefix, or Suffix
narrowing	-constriction
	-stenosis
nature	physi/o
navel	omphal/o
	umbilic/o
near	para-
	proxim/o
neck	cervic/o
neither	neutr/o
nerve	neur/o
nerve root	radicul/o
nest	nid/o
new	neo-
network	reticul/o
network of nerves	plex/o
neutral	neutr/o
night	noct/i
	nyct/o
nipple	thel/o
nipple-like	papill/o
nitrogen	azot/o
nitrogen compound	-amine
no, not	a-
	an-
none	nulli-
normal	eu-
nose	nas/o (use with -al)
	rhin/o (use with -itis, -rrhea, -plasty)
nourishment	troph/o
	-trophy
nucleus	kary/o
	nucle/o
nucleus (collection of nerve cells in the brain)	kern-
numbness	narc/o

English—Medical Word Parts *Continued*

Meaning	Combining Form, Prefix, or Suffix
obscure	-opaque
obsessive preoccupation	-mania
off	apo-
old age	ger/o
	presby/o
olecranon (elbow)	olecran/o
on	epi-
one	mon/o
	mono-
	uni-
one's own	aut/o
	auto-
one who	-er
	-or
opening	-tresia
opening (new)	-stomy
opposite	contra-
optic disc (disk)	papill/o
orange-yellow	cirrh/o
order	norm/o
	tax/o
organs, internal	viscer/o
ossicle	ossicul/o
other	all/o
other than	par-
out, outside	ec-
	ex-
	exo-
	extra-
outer region	cortic/o
ovary	oophor/o (use with -itis, -ectomy, -pexy)
	ovari/o (use with -an)
oxygen	ox/o
	-oxia

Chart continued on following page

English—Medical Word Parts *Continued*

Meaning	Combining Form, Prefix, or Suffix
pain	-algia
	-dynia
	odyn/o
pain, excessive	-agra
pain, sensitivity to	-algesia
	algesi/o
painful	dys-
palate	palat/o
palsy	-plegia
	-plegic
pancreas	pancreat/o
paralysis	-plegia
	-plegic
paralysis, slight	-paresis
patella	patell/a (use with -pexy)
	patell/o (use with -ar, -ectomy, -femoral)
pelvic bone, pelvis	pelv/i
	pelv/o
penis	balan/o
	phall/o
people	dem/o
perineum	perine/o
peritoneum	peritone/o
pertaining to	-ac (cardiac)
	-al (inguinal)
	-an (ovarian)
	-ar (palmar)
	-ary (papillary)
	-eal (pharyngeal)
	-iac (hypochondriac)
	-ic (nucleic)
	-ical (neurological)
	-ine (equine)

English—Medical Word Parts *Continued*

Meaning	Combining Form, Prefix, or Suffix
	-ior (superior)
	-ose (adipose)
	-ous (mucous)
	-tic (necrotic)
phalanges	phalang/o
pharynx (throat)	pharyng/o
phrase	-lexia
physician	iatr/o
pineal gland	pineal/o
pituitary gland	hypophys/o
	pituit/o
	pituitar/o
place	-stasis
	the/o
	top/o
plant	phyt/o
	-phyte
plaque	ather/o
	-plakia
pleura	pleur/o
pleural cavity	-thorax
plexus	plex/o
poison	tox/o
	toxic/o
pole	styl/o
polyp	polyp/o
pons	pont/o
pores (condition of)	-porosis
position	top/o
potassium	kal/i
pour	chym/o
	-fusion
pregnancy	-cyesis
	gest/o

Chart continued on following page

English—Medical Word Parts *Continued*

Meaning	Combining Form, Prefix, or Suffix
pregnancy	gester/o
	gravid/o
	-gravida
pressure	bar/o
	-tension
process	-ation
	-ion
	-ism
	-y
produced by or in	-genic
producing	-gen
	-genesis
prolapse	-ptosis
prostate gland	prostat/o
protection	immun/o
	-phylaxis
protein	-globin
	-globulin
	prote/o
pubis	pub/o
pulse	sphygm/o
	-sphyxia
puncture to remove fluid	-centesis
pupil	cor/o
	core/o
	pupill/o
pus	py/o, purul/o
put	the/o
put in place	-pexy
pyloric sphincter, pylorus	pylor/o
radioactivity	radi/o
radius (lower arm bone)	radi/o
rapid	oxy-

English—Medical Word Parts *Continued*

Meaning	Combining Form, Prefix, or Suffix
rash	exanthemat/o
rays	radi/o
record	-gram
recording, process of	-graphy
rectum	rect/o
recurring	cycl/o
red	erythr/o
redness	erythem/o
	erythemat/o
reduce	-lytic
relaxation	-chalasia, -chalasis
removal	-apheresis
	-ectomy
	-pheresis
renal pelvis	pyel/o
repair	-plasty
resembling	-form
	-oid
retina	retin/o
rib	cost/o
roll (to)	vol/o
rosy	eosin/o
round	spher/o
rule	norm/o
run	-drome
rupture	-rrhexis
sac, small	alveol/o
	follicul/o
sac of fluid	cyst/o
sacrum	sacr/o
safe	immun/o

Chart continued on following page

English—Medical Word Parts *Continued*

Meaning	Combining Form, Prefix, or Suffix
sag (to)	-ptosis
saliva	sial/o
salivary gland	sialaden/o
same	ipsi-
	is/o
sameness	home/o
scaly	ichthy/o
scanty	olig/o
sclera	scler/o
scrotum	scrot/o
sea	thalass/o
sebum	seb/o
	sebace/o
	steat/o
secrete	crin/o
	-crine
seed	gon/o
	semin/i
seizure	-lepsy
seize (to); take hold of	-leptic
self	aut/o
	auto-
semen	semin/i
seminal vesicle	vesicul/o
send (to)	-mission
sensation (nervous)	-esthesia
separate	-crine
separation	-lysis
set (to)	-stitial
severe	acu/o
sex glands	gonad/o
sexual intercourse	-pareunia
shape	-form
	morph/o
sharp	acu/o
	oxy-

English—Medical Word Parts *Continued*

Meaning	Combining Form, Prefix, or Suffix
sheath	thec/o
shield	thyr/o
shin bone	tibi/o
shine	-lucent
short	brachy-
shoulder	om/o
side	later/o
sieve	ethm/o
sigmoid colon	sigmoid/o
single	mon/o
sinus	sinus/o
skin	cutane/o (use with -ous)
	derm/o (use with -al)
	-derma (use with erythr/o, leuk/o)
	dermat/o (use with -itis, -logist, -logy, -osis)
	epitheli/o (use with -al, -lysis, -oid, -oma, -um)
skull	crani/o
sleep	hypn/o
	somn/o
	-somnia
sleep (deep)	comat/o
slender	lept/o
slide (to)	-lapse
	lux/o
slipping	-listhesis
slow	brady-
small	-icle
	micro-
	-ole
	-ule
small intestine	enter/o

Chart continued on following page

English—Medical Word Parts *Continued*

Meaning	Combining Form, Prefix, or Suffix
smaller	mi/o
smell	-osmia
sodium	natr/o
soft	medull/o
softening	-malacia
sole (of the foot)	plant/o
solution	-sol
sound	echo-
	phon/o
	-phonia
	son/o
spark	scint/i
specialist	-ist
speech	phas/o
	-phasia
sperm cells	sperm/o
(spermatozoa)	spermat/o
spinal column	rachi/o
spinal cord	myel/o
spinal column (spine)	spin/o
	rachi/o
	vertebr/o
spiny	acanth/o
spitting	-ptysis
spleen	splen/o
split	-fida
	schiz/o
split (to)	-schisis
stake (pole)	styl/o
stapes	staped/o
starch	amyl/o
state of	-sis
steal	klept/o
sternum	stern/o
steroid	ster/o

English—Medical Word Parts *Continued*

Meaning	Combining Form, Prefix, or Suffix
sticking together	agglutin/o
stiff	ankyl/o
stimulate	-tropin
stomach	gastr/o
stone	lith/o
stop	-suppression
stopping	-stasis
	-static
straight	orth/o
stranger	xen/o
strength	-sthenia
stretch	tone/o
stretching	-ectasia
	-ectasis
stricture	-stenosis
structure	-ium
	-um, -us
structure, solid	ster/o
study of	log/o
	-logy
stupor	narc/o
substance	-in
	-ine
substance that forms	-poietin
sudden	acu/o
	oxysm/o
sugar	gluc/o
	glyc/o
	glycos/o
	-ose
surgical repair	-plasty
surrounding	peri-
suture (to)	-rrhaphy
swallow	phag/o

Chart continued on following page

English—Medical Word Parts *Continued*

Meaning	Combining Form, Prefix, or Suffix
swallowing	-phagia
swayback	lord/o
sweat	diaphor/o (use with -esis)
	hidr/o (use with -osis)
swift	oxy-
sword	xiph/o
synovia (fluid)	synov/o
synovial membrane	synov/o
tail	caud/o
tailbone	coccyg/o
tear	dacry/o (use with -genic, -rrhea)
	lacrim/o (use with -al, -ation)
tear (to cut)	-spadia
tear gland	dacryoaden/o
tear sac	dacryocyst/o
temperament	cras/o
tendon	ten/o
	tend/o
	tendin/o
tension	ton/o
testis	orch/o (use with -itis)
	orchi/o (use with -algia, -dynia, -ectomy, -pathy, -pexy, -tomy)
	orchid/o (use with -ectomy, -pexy, -plasty, -ptosis, -tomy)
	test/o (use with -sterone)
thick	pachy-
thigh bone	femor/o
thin	lept/o

English—Medical Word Parts *Continued*

Meaning	Combining Form, Prefix, or Suffix
thing	-um
	-us
thirst	dips/o
thorny	acanth/o
three	tri-
throat	pharyng/o
through	dia-
	per-
	trans-
throw (to)	bol/o
thymus gland	thym/o
thyroid gland	thyr/o
	thyroid/o
tibia	tibi/o
tie	nect/o
tie together	-desis
tightening	-stenosis
time	chron/o
tissue	hist/o
	histi/o
	-ium
	-um
toes	dactyl/o
together	con-
	sym-
	syn-
tongue	gloss/o (use with -al, -dynia, -plasty, -plegia, -rrhaphy, -spasm, -tomy)
	lingu/o (use with -al)
tonsil	tonsill/o
tooth	dent/i
	odont/o
top	acr/o

Chart continued on following page

English—Medical Word Parts *Continued*

Meaning	Combining Form, Prefix, or Suffix
toward	ad-
	af-
trachea	trache/o
transmission	-phoresis
treatment	iatr/o
	therapeut/o
	-therapy
trigone	trigon/o
tube	syring/o
tumor	-oma
	onc/o
turn	-tropia
	-verse
	-version
turning	-tropic
twisted chains	strept/o
two	bi-
tympanic membrane	myring/o
	tympan/o
ulcer	aphth/o
ulna	uln/o
umbilicus, navel	omphal/o (use with -cele, -ectomy, -rrhagia, -rrhexis)
	umbilic/o (use with -al)
unchanging	home/o
under	hypo-
unequal	anis/o
unknown	idi/o
up	ana-
upon	epi-
urea	azot/o
ureter	ureter/o
urethra	urethr/o

English—Medical Word Parts *Continued*

Meaning	Combining Form, Prefix, or Suffix
urinary bladder	cyst/o (use with cele, -ectomy, -itis, -pexy, -plasty, -plegia, -scope, -scopy, -stomy, -tomy)
	vesic/o (use with -al)
urinary tract	ur/o
urination	-uria
urine	ur/o
	-uria
	urin/o
uterus	hyster/o (use with -ectomy, -graphy, -gram, -tomy)
	metr/o (use with -rrhagia, -rrhea, -rrhexis)
	metri/o (use with -osis)
	uter/o (use with -ine)
uvea	uve/o
uvula	uvul/o (use with -ar, -itis, -ptosis)
	staphyl/o (use with -ectomy, -plasty, -tomy)
vagina	colp/o (use with -pexy, -plasty, -scope, -scopy, -tomy)
	vagin/o (use with -al, -itis)
vagus nerve	vag/o
valve	valv/o
	valvul/o
varicose veins	varic/o
varied	poikil/o
vas deferens	vas/o

Chart continued on following page

English—Medical Word Parts *Continued*

Meaning	Combining Form, Prefix, or Suffix
vein	phleb/o (use with -ectomy, -itis, -tomy)
	ven/o (use with -ous, -gram)
vein, small	venul/o
ventricle	ventricul/o
vertebra	rachi/o (use with -itis, -tomy)
	spondyl/o (use with -itis, -listhesis, -osis, -pathy)
	vertebr/o (use with -al)
vessel	angi/o (use with -ectomy, -genesis, -gram, -graphy, -oma, -plasty, -spasm)
	vas/o (use with -constriction, -dilation, -motor)
	vascul/o (use with -ar, -itis)
view of	-opsy
vision	-opia
	-opsia
	opt/o
	optic/o
visual examination	-scopy
vitreous body	vitr/o
voice	phon/o
	-phonia
voice box	laryng/o
vomiting	-emesis
vulva	episi/o (use with -tomy)
	vulv/o (use with -ar)
wander	ion/o
washing	-clysis

English—Medical Word Parts Continued

Meaning	Combining Form, Prefix, or Suffix
wasting away	-phthisis
water	aque/o
	hydr/o
watery flow	rheumat/o
wedge	sphen/o
weight	bar/o
white	alb/o
	albin/o
	leuk/o
wide	mydr/o
widening	-dilation
	-ectasia
	-ectasis
	-eurysm
windpipe	trache/o
with	con-
	sym-
	syn-
within	en-
	endo-
	intra-
woman	gynec/o
womb	hyster/o
	metr/o
	metri/o
	uter/o
word	-lexia
work	erg/o
wrist bone	carp/o
x-rays	radi/o
yellow	lute/o
	jaund/o
	xanth/o

Abbreviations*

Many of these abbreviations may appear with or without periods and with either a capital or a lower-case first letter.

ā	before
A2 or A_2	aortic valve closure (heart sound)
AAA	abdominal aortic aneurysm
AAL	anterior axillary line
AB	abortion
ab	antibody
abd	abdomen; abduction
ABG	arterial blood gas
a.c.	before meals *(ante cibum)*
ACE	angiotensin-converting enzyme (ACE inhibitors are used to treat hypertension)
ACh	acetylcholine (neurotransmitter)
ACTH	adrenocorticotropic hormone (secreted by the anterior pituitary gland)
AD	right ear *(auris dextra);* Alzheimer disease
ADD	attention deficit disorder
add	adduction
ADH	antidiuretic hormone; vasopressin (secreted by the posterior pituitary gland)
ADHD	attention deficit hyperactivity disorder
ADL	activities of daily living
ADT	admission, discharge, transfer
ad lib	as desired
AF	atrial fibrillation

Chart continued on following page

---

*From Chabner DE: The Language of Medicine, 6th ed. Philadelphia, W.B. Saunders, 2001.

Abbreviations *Continued*

AFB	acid-fast bacillus (bacilli)
AFO	ankle foot orthosis (device for stabilization)
AFP	alpha-fetoprotein
AHF	antihemophilic factor (coagulation factor XIII)
AI	aortic insufficiency; artificial insemination
AIDS	acquired immunodeficiency syndrome
AIHA	autoimmune hemolytic anemia
AKA	above-knee amputation
alb	albumin (protein)
alk phos	alkaline phosphatase (elevated in liver disease)
ALL	acute lymphocytic leukemia
ALS	amyotrophic lateral sclerosis (Lou Gehrig disease)
ALT	alanine aminotransferase (elevated in liver and heart disease); formerly SGPT
Amb	ambulate, ambulatory (walking)
AML	acute myelocytic (myelogenous) leukemia
ANC	absolute neutrophil count
AODL	activities of daily living
AP, A.P., or A/P	anteroposterior
A&P	auscultation and percussion
aq.	water *(aqua);* aqueous
ARDS	adult respiratory distress syndrome
ARF	acute renal failure
ARMD	age-related macular degeneration
AROM	active range of motion
AS	left ear *(auris sinistra);* aortic stenosis
ASA	acetylsalicylic acid (aspirin)
ASD	atrial septal defect
ASH	asymmetrical septal hypertrophy
ASHD	arteriosclerotic heart disease
AST	aspartate aminotransferase (elevated in liver and heart disease); formerly SGOT

Abbreviations *Continued*

AU	both ears *(auris uterque)*
Au	gold
AV	arteriovenous; atrioventricular
AVM	arteriovenous malformation
AVR	aortic valve replacement
A&W	alive and well
Ba	barium
bands	banded neutrophils
baso	basophils
BBB	bundle branch block
BC	bone conduction
B cells	lymphocytes produced in the bone marrow
BE	barium enema
bid, b.i.d.	twice a day *(bis in die)*
BKA	below-knee amputation
BM	bowel movement
BMR	basal metabolic rate
BMT	bone marrow transplant
BP	blood pressure
BPH	benign prostatic hyperplasia (hypertrophy)
BRBPR	bright red blood per rectum; hematochezia
BSE	breast self-examination
BSO	bilateral salpingo-oophorectomy
BSP	Bromsulphalein (dye used in liver function test; its retention is indicative of liver damage or disease)
BT	bleeding time
BUN	blood urea nitrogen
Bx, bx	biopsy
C	Celsius or centigrade; calorie
c̄	with *(cum)*

Chart continued on following page

Abbreviations *Continued*

C1, C2	first, second cervical vertebra
CA	chronological age; cardiac arrest
Ca	calcium; cancer
CABG	coronary artery bypass graft
CAD	coronary artery disease
CAO	chronic airway obstruction
CAPD	continuous ambulatory peritoneal dialysis
cap	capsule
Cath	catheter; catheterization
CAT scan	computed (axial) tomography
CBC, c.b.c.	complete blood count
CC	chief complaint
cc	cubic centimeter (unit of volume; 1/1000 liter)
CCU	coronary care unit
CDH	congenital dislocated hip
CEA	carcinoembryonic antigen
cf.	compare
CF	cystic fibrosis
cGy	centigray (one hundredth of a gray; a rad)
CHD	coronary heart disease
chemo	chemotherapy
CHF	congestive heart failure
chol	cholesterol
chr	chronic
μCi	microcurie
CIN	cervical intraepithelial neoplasia
CIS	carcinoma *in situ*
CK	creatine kinase
Cl	chlorine
CLD	chronic liver disease
CLL	chronic lymphocytic leukemia
cm	centimeter (1/100 meter)
CMG	cystometrogram
CML	chronic myelogenous leukemia
CMV	cytomegalovirus
CNS	central nervous system

Abbreviations *Continued*

Co	cobalt
C/O	complains of
CO_2	carbon dioxide
COPD	chronic obstructive pulmonary disease
CP	cerebral palsy; chest pain
CPA	costophrenic angle
CPD	cephalopelvic disproportion
CPK	creatine phosphokinase
CPR	cardiopulmonary resuscitation
CR	complete response
CRF	chronic renal failure
CS	cesarean section
C&S	culture and sensitivity
C-section	cesarean section
CSF	cerebrospinal fluid
C-spine	cervical spine films
ct.	count
CTA	clear to auscultation
CTS	carpal tunnel syndrome
CT scan	computed tomography (x-ray images in a cross-sectional view)
CVA	cerebrovascular accident; costovertebral angle
CVP	central venous pressure
CVS	cardiovascular system; chorionic villus sampling
c/w	compare with; consistent with
CX (CXR)	chest x-ray
Cx	cervix
cysto	cystoscopy
D/C	discontinue; discharge
D&C	dilatation (dilation) and curettage
DCIS	ductal carcinoma *in situ*
DD	discharge diagnosis
Decub.	decubitus (lying down)
Derm.	dermatology

Chart continued on following page

Abbreviations *Continued*

DES	diethylstilbestrol; diffuse esophageal spasm
DI	diabetes insipidus; diagnostic imaging
DIC	disseminated intravascular coagulation
diff.	differential count (white blood cells)
DIG	digoxin; digitalis
dL, dl	deciliter (1/10 liter)
DLE	discoid lupus erythematosus
DM	diabetes mellitus
DNA	deoxyribonucleic acid
DNR	do not resuscitate
D.O.	Doctor of Osteopathy
DOA	dead on arrival
DOB	date of birth
DOE	dyspnea on exertion
DPT	diphtheria, pertussis, tetanus (vaccine)
DRE	digital rectal exam
DRG	diagnosis-related group
DSA	digital subtraction angiography
DSM	Diagnostic and Statistical Manual of Mental Disorders
DT	delirium tremens (caused by alcohol withdrawal)
DTR	deep tendon reflexes
DUB	dysfunctional uterine bleeding
DVT	deep venous thrombosis
Dx	diagnosis
EBV	Epstein-Barr virus
ECC	endocervical curettage; extracorporeal circulation
ECF	extended-care facility
ECG	electrocardiogram
ECHO	echocardiography
ECMO	extracorporeal membrane oxygenation
ECT	electroconvulsive therapy
ED	emergency department
EDC	estimated date of confinement

Abbreviations *Continued*

EEG	electroencephalogram
EENT	eyes, ears, nose, and throat
EGD	esophagogastroduodenoscopy
EKG	electrocardiogram
ELISA	enzyme-linked immunosorbent assay (AIDS test)
EM	electron microscope
EMB	endometrial biopsy
EMG	electromyogram
ENT	ear, nose, and throat
EOM	extraocular movement; extraocular muscles
eos.	eosinophil (type of white blood cell)
Epo	erythropoietin
ER	emergency room; estrogen receptor
ERCP	endoscopic retrograde cholangiopancreatography
ERT	estrogen replacement therapy
ESR	erythrocyte sedimentation rate
ESRD	end-stage renal disease
ESWL	extracorporeal shock wave lithotripsy
ETOH	ethyl alcohol
ETT	exercise tolerance test
F	Fahrenheit
FACP	Fellow, American College of Physicians
FACS	Fellow, American College of Surgeons
FB	fingerbreadth; foreign body
FBS	fasting blood sugar
FDA	Food and Drug Administration
Fe	iron
FEF	forced expiratory flow
FEV	forced expiratory volume
FH	family history
FHR	fetal heart rate
FROM	full range of movement/motion
FSH	follicle-stimulating hormone

Chart continued on following page

Abbreviations *Continued*

F/u	follow-up
5-FU	5-fluorouracil (used in cancer chemotherapy)
FUO	fever of undetermined origin
F_x, Fx	fracture
μg	microgram (one-millionth of a gram)
G	gravida (pregnant)
g, gm	gram
Ga	gallium
GABA	gamma-aminobutyric acid (neurotransmitter)
GB	gallbladder
GBS	gallbladder series (x-rays)
GC	gonorrhea
G-CSF	granulocyte colony-stimulating factor
GERD	gastroesophageal reflux disease
GFR	glomerular filtration rate
GH	growth hormone
GI	gastrointestinal
Grav. 1, 2, 3	first, second, third pregnancy
GTT	glucose tolerance test
gt, gtt	drop *(gutta)*, drops *(guttae)*
GU	genitourinary
Gy	gray (unit of radiation and equal to 100 rads)
GYN	gynecology
H	hydrogen
h, hr	hour
H2 blocker	H2 (histamine) receptor antagonist (inhibitor of gastric acid secretion)
HBV	hepatitis B virus
HCG (hCG)	human chorionic gonadotropin
HCl	hydrochloric acid

HCO₃	bicarbonate
Hct (HCT)	hematocrit
HCV	hepatitis C virus
HCVD	hypertensive cardiovascular disease
HD	hemodialysis (artificial kidney machine)
HDL	high-density lipoprotein
He	helium
HEENT	head, eyes, ears, nose, and throat
Hg	mercury
Hgb	hemoglobin
hGH	human growth hormone
H&H	hematocrit and hemoglobin
HIV	human immunodeficiency virus
HLA	histocompatibility locus antigen (identifies cells as "self")
HNP	herniated nucleus pulposus
h/o	history of
H₂O	water
hpf	high-power field (microscope)
HPI	history of present illness
HPV	human papillomavirus
HRT	hormone replacement therapy
h.s.	at bedtime *(hora somni)*
HSG	hysterosalpingography
HSV	herpes simplex virus
ht	height
HTN	hypertension (high blood pressure)
Hx	history
I	iodine
¹³¹I	radioactive isotope of iodine
IBD	inflammatory bowel disease
ICP	intracranial pressure
ICSH	interstitial cell-stimulating hormone
ICU	intensive care unit
I&D	incision and drainage

Chart continued on following page

Abbreviations *Continued*

ID	infectious disease
IDDM	insulin-dependent diabetes mellitus (type 1)
IgA, IgD, IgE, IgG, IgM	immunoglobulins
IHD	ischemic heart disease
IHSS	idiopathic hypertrophic subaortic stenosis
IM	intramuscular; infectious mononucleosis
IMV	intermittent mandatory ventilation
inf.	infusion; inferior
INH	isoniazid (drug used to treat tuberculosis)
inj.	injection
I&O	intake and output (measurement of patient's fluids)
IOL	intraocular lens (implant)
IOP	intraocular pressure
I.Q.	intelligence quotient
IUD	intrauterine device
IUP	intrauterine pregnancy
IV	intravenous (injection)
IVP	intravenous pyelogram
K	potassium
kg	kilogram (1000 grams)
KJ	knee jerk
KS	Kaposi sarcoma
KUB	kidney, ureter, and bladder (x-ray exam)
L, l	liter; left; lower
L1, L2	first, second lumbar vertebra
LA	left atrium
LAD	left anterior descending (coronary artery)

Abbreviations *Continued*

lat	lateral
LAVH	laparoscopic assisted vaginal hysterectomy
LB	large bowel
LBBB	left bundle branch block (heart block)
LD	lethal dose
LDH	lactate dehydrogenase (elevation associated with heart attacks)
LDL	low-density lipoprotein (high levels associated with heart disease)
L-dopa	levodopa (used to treat Parkinson disease)
L.E.	lupus erythematosus
LEEP	loop electrocautery excision procedure
LES	lower esophageal sphincter
LFTs	liver function tests
LH	luteinizing hormone
LLL	left lower lobe (lung)
LLQ	left lower quadrant (abdomen)
LMP	last menstrual period
LOC	loss of consciousness
LOS	length of stay
LP	lumbar puncture
lpf	low power field (microscope)
LPN	licensed practical nurse
LS	lumbosacral spine
LSD	lysergic acid diethylamide
LSK	liver, spleen, and kidneys
LTB	laryngotracheal bronchitis
LTC	long-term care
LTH	luteotropic hormone (prolactin)
LUL	left upper lobe (lung)
LUQ	left upper quadrant (abdomen)
LV	left ventricle
L&W	living and well
lymphs	lymphocytes
lytes	electrolytes

Chart continued on following page

MA	mental age
MAI	*Mycobacterium avium intracellulare*
MAOI	monoamine oxidase inhibitor (antidepressant drug)
MBD	minimal brain dysfunction
mcg	microgram
MCH	mean corpuscular hemoglobin (average amount in each red blood cell)
MCHC	mean corpuscular hemoglobin concentration (average concentration in a single red cell)
mCi	millicurie
μCi	microcurie
MCP	metacarpophalangeal joint
MCV	mean corpuscular volume (average size of a single red blood cell)
M.D.	Doctor of Medicine
MED	minimum effective dose
mEq	milliequivalent
mEq/L	milliequivalent per liter (measurement of the concentration of a solution)
mets	metastases
Mg	magnesium
mg	milligram (1/1000 gram)
mg/cc	milligram per cubic centimeter
mg/dl	milligram per deciliter
μg	microgram (one-millionth of a gram)
MH	marital history; mental health
MI	myocardial infarction; mitral insufficiency
mL, ml	milliliter (1/1000 liter)
mm	millimeter (1/1000 meter; 0.039 inch)
mmHg	millimeters of mercury
MMPI	Minnesota Multiphasic Personality Inventory
MMR	measles-mumps-rubella (vaccine)
MMT	manual muscle testing
mμ	millimicron (1/1000 micron; a micron is 10^{-3} mm)

Abbreviations *Continued*

μm	micrometer (one-millionth of a meter)
mono	monocyte (white blood cell)
MR	mitral regurgitation
MRI	magnetic resonance imaging
mRNA	messenger RNA
MS	multiple sclerosis; mitral stenosis
MSL	midsternal line
MTX	methotrexate
MUGA	multiple-gated acquisition scan (of heart)
multip	multipara; multiparous
MVP	mitral valve prolapse
N	nitrogen
Na	sodium
NB	newborn
NBS	normal bowel or breath sounds
ND	normal delivery; normal development
NED	no evidence of disease
neg.	negative
NG tube	nasogastric tube
NHL	non-Hodgkin lymphoma
NIDDM	non−insulin-dependent diabetes mellitus (type 2)
NK cells	natural killer cells
NKDA	no known drug allergies
NPO	nothing by mouth *(non per os)*
NSAID	nonsteroidal anti-inflammatory drug
NSR	normal sinus rhythm (of heart)
NTP	normal temperature and pressure
O	oxygen
OA	osteoarthritis
OB/GYN	obstetrics and gynecology
OCPs	oral contraceptive pills
O.D.	Doctor of Optometry; overdose; right eye *(oculus dexter)*

Chart continued on following page

Abbreviations *Continued*

OR	operating room
ORIF	open reduction internal fixation
ORTH; Ortho.	orthopedics
O.S.	left eye *(oculus sinister)*
os	opening; mouth; bone
O.T.	occupational therapy
O.U.	each eye *(oculus uterque)*
oz.	ounce
P	phosphorus; posterior; pressure; pulse; pupil
$\bar{p}$	after
P2 or P_2	pulmonary valve closure (heart sound)
PA	pulmonary artery; posteroanterior
P-A	posteroanterior
P&A	percussion and auscultation
PAC	premature atrial contraction
$PaCO_2$, pCO_2	partial pressure of carbon dioxide (in blood)
palp.	palpable; palpation
PALS	pediatric advanced life support
PaO_2, pO_2	partial pressure of oxygen
Pap smear	Papanicolaou smear (cells from cervix and vagina)
Para 1, 2, 3	unipara, bipara, tripara (number of viable births)
p.c.	after meals *(post cibum)*
PCP	*Pneumocystis carinii* pneumonia; phencyclidine (hallucinogen)
PCR	polymerase chain reaction (process allows making copies of genes)
PD	peritoneal dialysis
PDA	patent ductus arteriosus
PDR	Physicians' Desk Reference
PE	physical examination; pulmonary embolism
PEEP	positive end-expiratory pressure

Abbreviations *Continued*

PEG	percutaneous endoscopic gastrostomy (a feeding tube)
PEJ	percutaneous endoscopic jejunostomy (a feeding tube)
per os	by mouth
PERRLA	pupils equal, round, react to light and accommodation
PET	positron emission tomography
PE tube	ventilating tube for eardrum
PFT	pulmonary function test
PG	prostaglandin
PH	past history
pH	hydrogen ion concentration (alkalinity and acidity measurement)
PI	present illness
PID	pelvic inflammatory disease
PIP	proximal interphalangeal joint
PKU	phenylketonuria
p.m.	afternoon (post meridian)
PMH	past medical history
PMN	polymorphonuclear leukocyte
PMS	premenstrual syndrome
PND	paroxysmal nocturnal dyspnea
p/o	postoperative
p.o.	by mouth *(per os)*
poly	polymorphonuclear leukocyte
postop	postoperative (after surgery)
PPBS	postprandial blood sugar
PPD	purified protein derivative (test for tuberculosis)
preop	preoperative
prep	prepare for
PR	partial response
primip	primipara
PRL	prolactin
p.r.n.	as required *(pro re nata)*
procto	proctoscopy
prot.	protocol

Chart continued on following page

Abbreviations *Continued*

Pro. time	prothrombin time (test of blood clotting)
PSA	prostate-specific antigen
PT	prothrombin time; physical therapy
PTA	prior to admission (to hospital)
PTC	percutaneous transhepatic cholangiography
PTCA	percutaneous transluminal coronary angioplasty
PTH	parathyroid hormone
PTT	partial thromboplastin time (test of blood clotting)
PU	pregnancy urine
PUVA therapy	psoralen ultraviolet A (treatment for psoriasis)
PVC	premature ventricular contraction
PVD	peripheral vascular disease
PWB	partial weight bearing

q	every *(quaque)*
q.d.	every day *(quaque die)*
q.h.	every hour *(quaque hora)*
q.i.d.	four times daily *(quater in die)*
q.n.	each night *(quaque nox)*
q.s.	as much as suffices *(quantum sufficit)*
qt	quart

R	respiration; right
RA	rheumatoid arthritis; right atrium
Ra	radium
rad	radiation absorbed dose
RBBB	right bundle branch block
RBC, rbc	red blood cell (corpuscle); red blood count
R.D.D.A.	recommended daily dietary allowance
RDS	respiratory distress syndrome
REM	rapid eye movement

Abbreviations *Continued*

RF	rheumatoid factor
Rh	rhesus (monkey) factor in blood
RIA	radioimmunoassay (minute quantities are measured)
RIND	reversible ischemic neurologic deficit/defect
RLL	right lower lobe (lung)
RLQ	right lower quadrant (abdomen)
RML	right middle lobe (lung)
RNA	ribonucleic acid
R/O	rule out
ROM	range of motion
ROS	review of systems
RRR	regular rate and rhythm (of the heart)
RT	right; radiation therapy
RUL	right upper lobe (lung)
RUQ	right upper quadrant (abdomen)
RV	right ventricle
Rx	treatment; therapy; prescription
$\bar{s}$	without *(sine)*
S1, S2	first, second sacral vertebra
S-A node	sinoatrial node (pacemaker of heart)
SAD	seasonal affective disorder
SBE	subacute bacterial endocarditis
SBFT	small bowel follow-through (x-rays of small intestine)
sed. rate	sedimentation rate (rate of erythrocyte sedimentation)
segs	segmented neutrophils; polys
SERM	selective estrogen receptor modifier
SGOT (AST)	serum glutamic-oxaloacetic transaminase
SGPT (ALT)	serum glutamic-pyruvic transaminase
SIADH	syndrome of inappropriate antidiuretic hormone

Chart continued on following page

Abbreviations *Continued*

SIDS	sudden infant death syndrome
sig.	let it be labeled
SLE	systemic lupus erythematosus
SMA 12	twelve blood chemistries
SOAP	subjective, objective, assessment, and plan
SOB	shortness of breath
s.o.s.	if necessary *(si opus sit)*
S/P	status post (previous disease condition)
SPECT	single-photon emission computed tomography
sp. gr.	specific gravity
SSRI	selective serotonin reuptake inhibitor (antidepressant)
Staph.	staphylococci (berry-shaped bacteria in clusters)
stat.	immediately *(statim)*
STD	sexually transmitted disease
STH	somatotropin (growth hormone)
Strep.	streptococci (berry-shaped bacteria in twisted chains)
Subcu	subcutaneous
SVC	superior vena cava
SVD	spontaneous vaginal delivery
Sx	symptoms
T	temperature; time
T1, T2	first, second thoracic vertebra
T_3	triiodothyronine
T_4	thyroxine
TA	therapeutic abortion
T&A	tonsillectomy and adenoidectomy
TAH	total abdominal hysterectomy
TAT	Thematic Apperception Test
TB	tuberculosis
Tc	technetium
T cells	lymphocytes produced in the thymus gland

TEE	transesophageal echocardiogram
TENS	transcutaneous electrical nerve stimulation
TFT	thyroid function test
TIA	transient ischemic attack
t.i.d.	three times daily *(ter in die)*
TLC	total lung capacity
TM	tympanic membrane
TMJ	temporomandibular joint
TNM	tumor, nodes, and metastases
tPA	tissue plasminogen activator
TPN	total parenteral nutrition
TPR	temperature, pulse, and respiration
TRUS	transrectal ultrasound
TSH	thyroid-stimulating hormone
TSS	toxic shock syndrome
TUR, TURP	transurethral resection of the prostate
TVH	total vaginal hysterectomy
Tx	treatment
U	unit
UA	urinalysis
UAO	upper airway obstruction
UC	uterine contractions
UE	upper extremity
UGI	upper gastrointestinal
umb.	navel *(umbilicus)*
U/O	urinary output
URI	upper respiratory infection
U/S	ultrasound
UTI	urinary tract infection
UV	ultraviolet
VA	visual acuity
VC	vital capacity (of lungs)

Chart continued on following page

Abbreviations *Continued*

VCUG	voiding cystourethrogram
VF	visual field
vis à vis	as compared with; in relation to
V/Q scan	ventilation-perfusion scan
V/S	vital signs; versus
VSD	ventricular septal defect
VT	ventricular tachycardia (abnormal heart rhythm)
WAIS	Wechsler Adult Intelligence Scale
WBC, wbc	white blood cell; white blood count
WDWN	well developed, well nourished
WISC	Wechsler Intelligence Scale for Children
WNL	within normal limits
wt	weight
XRT	radiation therapy
y/o, yrs	year(s) old

Symbols*

=	equal
≠	unequal
+	positive
−	negative
↑	above, increase
↓	below, decrease
♀	female
♂	male
→	to (in direction of)
>	is greater than
<	is less than
1°	primary to
2°	secondary to
ℨ	dram
℥	ounce
%	percent
°	degree; hour
:	ratio; "is to"
±	plus or minus (either positive or negative)
′	foot
″	inch
∴	therefore
@	at, each
c̄	with
s̄	without
#	pound
≅	approximately, about
Δ	change
p	short arm of a chromosome
q	long arm of a chromosome

* From Chabner DE: The Language of Medicine, 6th ed. Philadelphia, W.B. Saunders, 2001.

Plurals*

The rules commonly used to form plurals of medical terms are as follows:

1. For words ending in a, retain the a and add e: Examples:

Singular	*Plural*
vertebra	vertebrae
bursa	bursae
bulla	bullae

2. For words ending in is, drop the is and add es: Examples:

Singular	*Plural*
anastomosis	anastomoses
metastasis	metastases
epiphysis	epiphyses
prosthesis	prostheses
pubis	pubes

3. For words ending in ix and ex, drop the ix or ex and add ices: Examples:

Singular	*Plural*
apex	apices
varix	varices

4. For words ending in on, drop the on and add a: Examples:

Singular	*Plural*
ganglion	ganglia
spermatozoon	spermatozoa

---

*From Chabner DE: The Language of Medicine, 6th ed. Philadelphia, W.B. Saunders, 2001.

5. For words ending in **um**, drop the **um** and add **a**:
Examples:

Singular	Plural
bacterium	bacteria
diverticulum	diverticula
ovum	ova

6. For words ending in **us**, drop the **us** and add **i**:
Examples:

Singular	Plural
calculus	calculi
bronchus	bronchi
nucleus	nuclei

Two exceptions to this rule are viruses and sinuses.

7. Examples of other plural changes are:

Singular	Plural
foramen	foramina
iris	irides
femur	femora
anomaly	anomalies
biopsy	biopsies
adenoma	adenomata

Definitions of Diagnostic Tests and Procedures*

Radiology, Ultrasound, and Imaging Procedures

In many of the following procedures a *contrast* substance (sometimes referred to as a *dye*) is introduced into or around a body part so that the part can be viewed while x-rays are taken. The contrast substance (often containing barium or iodine) appears dense on the x-ray and outlines the body part that it fills.

The suffix -GRAPHY, meaning "process of recording," is used in many terms describing imaging procedures. The suffix -GRAM, meaning "record," is also used and describes the actual image that is produced by the procedure.

Pronunciation of each term is given with its meaning. The syllable that gets the accent is in CAPITAL LETTERS. Terms in SMALL CAPITAL LETTERS are defined elsewhere in the appendix.

ANGIOGRAPHY (an-je-OG-rah-fe) or ANGIOGRAM (AN-je-o-gram): X-ray recording of blood vessels. A contrast substance is injected into blood vessels (veins and arteries), and x-ray pictures are taken of the vessels. In *cerebral angiography,* x-ray pictures are taken of blood vessels in the brain. Angiography is used to detect abnormalities in blood vessels, such as blockage, malformation, and arteriosclerosis. Angiography is performed most frequently to view arteries and is often used interchangeable with *arteriography.*

---

* From Chabner DE: Medical Terminology: A Short Course, 2nd ed. Philadelphia, W.B. Saunders, 1999.

ARTERIOGRAPHY (ar-ter-e-OG-rah-fe) or ARTERIO-GRAM (ar-TER-e-oh-gram): X-ray recording of arteries after injection of a contrast substance into an artery. *Coronary arteriography* is the visualization of arteries that bring blood to the heart muscle.

BARIUM TESTS (BAR-re-um tests): X-ray examinations using a liquid barium mixture to locate disorders in the esophagus *(esophagogram),* duodenum, small intestine *(small bowel follow through),* and colon *(barium enema).* Taken before or during the examination, barium causes the intestinal tract to stand out in silhouette when viewed through a *fluoroscope* or seen on an x-ray film. The *barium swallow* is used to examine the upper gastrointestinal tract, and the *barium enema* is for examination of the lower gastrointestinal tract.

BARIUM ENEMA: See LOWER GASTROINTESTINAL EXAMINATION AND BARIUM TESTS.

BARIUM SWALLOW: See ESOPHAGOGRAPHY AND BARIUM TESTS.

CARDIAC CATHETERIZATION (KAR-de-ak cath-eh-ter-i-ZA-shun): A catheter (tube) is passed via vein or artery into the chambers of the heart. This procedure is used to measure the blood flow out of the heart and the pressures and oxygen content in the heart chambers. Contrast material is also introduced into heart chambers and x-ray images are taken to show heart structure.

CT SCAN, CAT SCAN: X-ray images are taken to show the body in cross-section. Contrast material may be used (injected into the bloodstream) to highlight structures such as the liver, brain, or blood vessels, and barium can be swallowed to outline gastrointestinal organs. X-ray images, taken as the x-ray tube rotates around the body, are processed by a computer to show "slices" of body tissues, most often within the head, chest, and abdomen.

CEREBRAL ANGIOGRAPHY: See ANGIOGRAPHY.

CHEST X-RAY: An x-ray of the chest may show infection (as in pneumonia or tuberculosis), emphysema, occupational exposure (asbestosis), lung tumors, or heart enlargement.

CHOLANGIOGRAPHY (kol-an-je-OG-rah-fe) or CHOLANGIOGRAM (kol-an-je-o-gram): X-ray recording of bile ducts. Contrast material is given by intravenous injection *(IV cholangiogram)* and collects in the gallbladder and bile ducts or is directly inserted by a tube through the mouth into bile ducts *(T-tube cholangiogram)*. X-rays are taken of bile ducts to identify obstructions caused by tumors or stones.

CORONARY ARTERIOGRAPHY: See ARTERIOGRAPHY.

CYSTOGRAPHY (sis-TOG-rah-fe) or CYSTOGRAM (SIS-to-gram): X-ray recording of the urinary bladder using a contrast medium, so that the outline of the urinary bladder can be seen clearly. A contrast substance is injected via catheter into the urethra and urinary bladder, and x-ray images are taken. A *voiding cystourethrogram* is an x-ray image of the urinary tract made while the patient is urinating.

DIGITAL SUBTRACTION ANGIOGRAPHY (DIJ-i-tal sub-TRAK-shun an-je-OG-rah-fe): A unique x-ray technique for viewing blood vessels by taking two images and subtracting one from the other. Images are first taken without contrast and then again after contrast is injected into blood vessels. The first image is then subtracted from the second so that the final image (sharp and precise) shows only contrast-filled blood vessels minus surrounding tissue.

ECHOCARDIOGRAPHY (eh-ko-kar-de-OG-rah-fe) or ECHOCARDIOGRAM (eh-ko-KAR-de-o-gram): Images of the heart are produced by introducing high-frequency sound waves through the chest into the heart. The sound waves are reflected back from the heart, and echoes showing heart structure are displayed on a recording machine. It is a highly useful diagnostic tool in the evaluation of diseases of the valves that separate the heart chambers and diseases of the heart muscle.

ECHOENCEPHALOGRAPHY (eh-ko-en-sef-ah-LOG-rah-fe) or ECHOENCEPHALOGRAM (eh-ko-en-SEF-ah-lo-gram): An ultrasound recording of the brain. Sound waves are beamed at the brain, and the echoes that return to the machine are recorded as graphic tracings. Brain tumors and hematomas can be detected by abnormal tracings.

ENDOSCOPIC RETROGRADE CHOLANGIOPANCRE-ATOGRAPHY (en-do-SKOP-ik REH-tro-grad kol-an-je-o-pan-kre-ah-TOG-rah-fe): X-ray recording of the bile ducts, pancreas, and pancreatic duct. Contrast is injected via a tube through the mouth into the bile and pancreatic ducts and x-rays are then taken.

ESOPHAGOGRAPHY (eh-sof-ah-GOG-rah-fe) or ESOPH-AGOGRAM (eh-SOF-ah-go-gram): Barium sulfate is swallowed and x-ray images are taken of the esophagus. This test is also called a *barium meal* or *barium swallow* and is part of an *upper gastro-intestinal examination.*

FLUOROSCOPY (flur-OS-ko-pe): An x-ray procedure that uses a fluorescent screen rather than a photographic plate to show images of the body. X-rays that have passed through the body strike a screen covered with a fluorescent substance that emits yellow-green light. Internal organs are seen directly and in motion. Fluoroscopy is used to guide the insertion of catheters and during *barium tests.*

GALLBLADDER ULTRASOUND (gawl-BLA-der UL-tra-sownd): Sound waves are used to visualize gallstones. This procedure has replaced cholecys-tography, which required ingesting an iodine-based contrast substance.

HYSTEROSALPINGOGRAPHY (his-ter-o-sal-ping-OG-rah-fe) or HYSTEROSALPINGOGRAM (his-ter-o-sal-PING-o-gram): X-ray recording of the uterus and fallopian tubes. Contrast medium is inserted through the vagina into the uterus and fallopian tubes, and x-rays are taken to detect blockage or tumor.

INTRAVENOUS PYELOGRAPHY: See UROGRAPHY.

LOWER GASTROINTESTINAL EXAMINATION (LOwer gas-tro-in-TES-tin-al ek-zam-ih-NA-shun): A liquid contrast substance called barium sulfate is inserted through a plastic tube (enema) into the rectum and large intestine (colon). X-ray pictures of the colon are then taken. If tumor is present in the colon, it may appear as an obstruction or irregularity. Also known as a *barium enema.*

LYMPHANGIOGRAPHY (limf-an-je-OG-rah-fe) or LYMPHANGIOGRAM (limf-AN-je-o-gram): X-ray recording of lymph nodes and lymph vessels after contrast is injected into lymphatic vessels in the feet. The contrast medium travels upward through the lymphatic vessels of the pelvis, abdomen, and chest and outlines the architecture of lymph nodes in all areas of the body. This procedure is used to detect tumors within the lymphatic system. It is also known as *lymphography.*

LYMPHOGRAPHY: See LYMPHANGIOGRAPHY.

MAGNETIC RESONANCE IMAGING (mag-NET-ik REZ-o-nans IM-a-jing): Magnetic waves and radiofrequency pulses, not x-rays, are used to create an image of body organs. The images can be taken in several planes of the body—frontal, sagittal (side), and transverse (cross-section)—and are particularly useful for studying brain tumors and tumors of the chest cavity. This procedure is also known as an *MRI.*

MAMMOGRAPHY (mah-MOG-rah-fe) or MAMMOGRAM (MAM-o-gram): X-ray recording of the breast. X-rays of low voltage are beamed at the breast and images are produced. Mammography is used to detect abnormalities in breast tissue, such as early breast cancer.

MYELOGRAPHY (mi-eh-LOG-rah-fe) or MYELOGRAM (MI-eh-lo-gram): X-ray recording of the spinal cord. X-rays are taken of the fluid-filled space surrounding the spinal cord after a contrast medium is injected into the subarachnoid space (between the membranes surrounding the spinal cord) at the lumbar level of the back. Myelography detects tumors or ruptured, "slipped," discs (disks) that lie between the backbones (vertebrae) and press on the spinal cord.

PYELOGRAPHY or PYELOGRAM: See UROGRAPHY.

SMALL BOWEL FOLLOW-THROUGH: See BARIUM TESTS AND UPPER GASTROINTESTINAL EXAMINATION.

TOMOGRAPHY (to-MOG-rah-fe) or TOMOGRAM (TO-mo-gram): X-ray recording that shows an organ in depth. Several pictures ("slices") are taken of an organ by moving the x-ray tube and film in sequence to blur out certain regions and bring others into sharper focus. Tomograms of the kidney and lung are examples.

ULTRASONOGRAPHY (ul-tra-so-NOG-rah-fe) or UL-TRASONOGRAM (ul-tra-SON-o-gram): Images are produced by beaming sound waves into the body and capturing the echoes that bounce off organs. These echoes are then processed to produce an image, not in the sharpest detail, but showing the difference between fluid and solid masses and the general position of organs.

UPPER GASTROINTESTINAL EXAMINATION (UP-er gas-tro-in-TES-tin-al ek-zam-ih-NA-shun): A liquid contrast substance called barium sulfate is swallowed and x-ray pictures are taken of the esophagus *(barium meal* or *barium swallow),* duo-denum, and small intestine. In a *small bowel fol-low-through,* pictures are taken at increasing time intervals to follow the progress of barium through the small intestine. Identification of obstructions or ulcers is possible.

UROGRAPHY (u-ROG-rah-fe) or UROGRAM (UR-o-gram): X-ray recording of the kidney and urinary tract. If x-rays are taken after contrast medium is injected intravenously, the procedure is called *in-travenous urography (descending* or *excretion urography)* or *intravenous pyelography (IVP).* If x-rays are taken after injection of contrast medium into the bladder through the urethra, the procedure is *retrograde urography* or *retrograde pyelography*. Pyel/o means renal pelvis (the collecting chamber of the kidney).

Nuclear Medicine Scans

In the following diagnostic tests, radioactive material *(radioisotope)* is injected, inhaled, or swallowed and then detected by a scanning device in the organ in which it accumulates. X-rays, ultrasound, or magnetic waves are not used.

Pronunciation of each term is given with its meaning. The syllable that gets the accent is in CAPITAL LETTERS.

BONE SCAN (bon skan): A radioactive substance is injected intravenously, and its uptake in bones is detected by a scanning device. Tumors in bone can be detected by increased uptake of the radioactive material in the areas of the lesions.

BRAIN SCAN (bran skan): A radioactive substance is injected intravenously and collects in any lesion that disturbs the natural barrier that exists between blood vessels and normal brain tissue (blood-brain barrier), allowing the radioactive substance to enter the brain tissue. A scanning device detects the presence of the radioactive substance and thus can identify an area of tumor, abscess, or hematoma.

GALLIUM SCAN (GAL-le-um skan): Radioactive gallium (gallium citrate) is injected into the bloodstream and is detected in the body using a scanning device that produces an image of the areas where gallium collects. The gallium collects in areas of certain tumors (Hodgkin disease, hepatoma, various adenocarcinomas) and in areas of infection.

POSITRON EMISSION TOMOGRAPHY (POS-i-tron e-MISH-un to-MOG-rah-fe): Radioactive substances (oxygen and glucose are used) that release radioactive particles called positrons are injected into the body and travel to specialized areas such as the brain and heart. Because of the way that the positrons are released, cross-sectional color pictures can be made showing the location of the radioactive substance. This test is used to study disorders of the brain and to diagnose strokes, epilepsy, schizophrenia, and migraine headaches. Also known as a *PET scan.*

PULMONARY PERFUSION SCAN (PUL-mon-ar-e per-FU-shun skan): Radioactive particles are injected intravenously and travel rapidly to areas of the lung that are adequately filled with blood. Regions of obstructed blood flow due to tumor, blood clot, swelling, and inflammation can be seen as nonradioactive areas on the scan.

PULMONARY VENTILATION SCAN (PUL-mon-ar-e ven-ti-LA-shun skan): Radioactive gas (xenon-133) is inhaled, and a special camera detects its presence in the lungs. The scan is used to detect lung segments that fail to fill with the radioactive gas. Lack of filling is usually due to diseases that obstruct the bronchial tubes and air sacs. This scan is also used in the evaluation of lung function prior to surgery.

MYOCARDIAL SCAN (mi-o-KAR-de-al skan): A radioactive substance (thallium chloride-201) is injected intravenously and travels to the heart muscle while the patient is at rest or exercising. A special camera shows up areas that have inadequate collection of radioactive substance, such as areas of blocked blood vessels.

THYROID SCAN (THI-royd skan): A radioactive iodine chemical is injected intravenously and collects in the thyroid gland. A scanning device detects the radioactive substance in the gland, measuring it and producing an image of the gland. The increased or decreased activity of the gland is demonstrated by the gland's capacity to use the radioactive iodine. A thyroid scan is used to evaluate the position, size, and functioning of the thyroid gland.

Clinical Procedures

The following procedures are performed on patients to establish a correct diagnosis of an abnormal condition. In some instances, the procedure may also be used to treat the condition.

Pronunciation of each term is given with its meaning. The syllable that gets the accent is in CAPITAL LETTERS. Terms in SMALL CAPITAL LETTERS are defined elsewhere in the appendix.

ABDOMINOCENTESIS (ab-dom-in-o-sen-TE-sis): See PARACENTESIS.

AMNIOCENTESIS (am-ne-o-sen-TE-sis): Surgical puncture to remove fluid from the sac (amnion) that surrounds the fetus in the uterus. The fluid contains cells from the fetus that can be examined under a microscope.

ASPIRATION (as-peh-RA-shun): The withdrawal of fluid by suction through a needle or tube. The term "aspiration pneumonia" refers to an infection caused by inhalation into the lungs of food or an object.

AUDIOGRAM (AW-de-o-gram): A test using sound waves of various frequencies (e.g., 500 Hz up to 8000 Hz), which quantify the extent and type of hearing loss.

AUSCULTATION (aw-skul-TA-shun): The process of listening for sounds produced within the body. This is most often performed with the aid of a stethoscope to determine the condition of the chest or abdominal organs or to detect the fetal heart beat.

BIOPSY (BI-op-se): The removal of a piece of tissue from the body and subsequent examination of the tissue under a microscope. The procedure is performed by means of a surgical knife, needle aspiration, or via endoscopic removal (using a special forceps-like instrument inserted through a hollow flexible tube.) An *excisional biopsy* means that the entire tissue to be examined is removed. An *inci-*

sional biopsy is the removal of only a small amount of tissue, and a *needle biopsy* indicates that tissue is pierced with a hollow needle and fluid is withdrawn for microscopic examination.

BONE MARROW BIOPSY (bon MAH-ro BI-op-se): The removal of a small amount of bone marrow. The cells are then examined under a microscope. Often the hip bone (iliac crest) is used, and the biopsy is helpful in determining the number and type of blood cells in the bone marrow.

BRONCHOSCOPY (brong-KOS-ko-pe): The insertion of a flexible tube (endoscope) into the airway. The lining of the bronchial tubes can be seen, and tissue may be removed for biopsy. The tube is usually inserted through the mouth, but can also be directly inserted into the airway during *mediastinoscopy*. Sedation is required for this procedure.

COLONOSCOPY (ko-lon-OS-ko-pe): The insertion of a flexible tube (endoscope) through the rectum into the colon for visual examination. Biopsy samples may be taken and benign growths, such as polyps, can be removed through the endoscope. The removal of a polyp is called a polypectomy (pol-eh-PEK-to-me).

COLPOSCOPY (kol-POS-ko-pe): The inspection of the cervix through the insertion of a special microscope into the vagina. The vaginal walls are held apart by a speculum so that the cervix (entrance to the uterus) can come into view.

CONIZATION (ko-nih-ZA-shun): The removal of a cone-shaped sample of uterine cervix tissue. This sample is then examined under a microscope for evidence of cancerous growth. The special shape of the tissue sample allows the pathologist to examine the transitional zone of the cervix where cancers are most likely to develop.

CULDOCENTESIS (kul-do-sen-TE-sis): The insertion of a thin, hollow, needle through the vagina into the cul-de-sac, the space between the rectum and the uterus. Fluid is withdrawn and analyzed for evidence of cancerous cells, infection, or blood cells.

CYSTOSCOPY (sis-TOS-ko-pe): The insertion of a thin tube or cystoscope (endoscope) into the ure-thra and then into the urinary bladder in order to visualize the bladder. A biopsy of the urinary blad-der can be performed through the cystoscope.

DIGITAL RECTAL EXAMINATION (DIG-ih-tal REK-tal eks-am-ih-NA-shun): Physician inserts a gloved finger into the rectum. This procedure is used to detect rectal cancer and as a primary method of detection of prostate cancer.

DILATION AND CURETTAGE (di-LA-shun and kur-ih-TAJ): A series of probes of increasing size are systematically inserted through the vagina into the opening of the cervix. The cervix is thus dilated (widened) so that a curette (spoon-shaped instru-ment) can be inserted to remove tissue from the lining of the uterus. The tissue is then examined under a microscope. The abbreviation for this pro-cedure is *D and C.*

ELECTROCARDIOGRAPHY (e-lek-tro-kar-de-OG-rah-fe): The connection of electrodes (wires or "leads") to the body to record electric impulses from the heart. The *electrocardiogram* is the ac-tual record produced, and it is useful in discover-ing abnormalities in heart rhythms and diagnosing heart disorders. Abbreviation is *EKG or ECG.*

ELECTROENCEPHALOGRAPHY (e-lek-tro-en-sef-ah-LOG-rah-fe): The connection of electrodes (wires or "leads") to the scalp to record electricity com-ing from within the brain. The *electroencephalo-gram* is the actual record produced. It is useful in the diagnosis and monitoring of epilepsy and other brain lesions and in the investigation of neurologi-cal disorders. It is also used to evaluate patients in coma (brain inactivity) and in the study of sleep disorders. Abbreviation is *EEG.*

ELECTROMYOGRAPHY (e-lek-tro-mi-OG-rah-fe): The insertion of needle electrodes into muscle to record electrical activity. This procedure detects injuries and diseases that affect muscles and nerves. Abbreviation is *EMG.*

ENDOSCOPY (en-DOS-ko-pe): The insertion of a thin, tube-like instrument (endoscope) into an organ or cavity. The endoscope is placed through a natural opening (the mouth or anus), or into a surgical incision, as through the abdominal wall. Endoscopes contain bundles of glass fibers that carry light (fiberoptic); some instruments are equipped with a small forceps-like device that withdraws a sample of tissue for microscopic study (biopsy). Examples of endoscopy are *bronchoscopy, colonoscopy, esophagoscopy, gastroscopy,* and *laparoscopy.*

ESOPHAGOSCOPY (eh-sof-ah-GOS-ko-pe): The insertion of an endoscope through the mouth and throat into the esophagus. Visual examination of the esophagus to detect ulcers, tumors, or other lesions is thus possible.

ESOPHAGOGASTRODUODENOSCOPY (eh-SOF-ah-go-GAS-tro-du-o-den-NOS-ko-pe): An endoscope is inserted through the mouth into the esophagus, stomach and first part of the small intestine. Also called *EGD.*

EXCISIONAL BIOPSY (ek-SIZ-in-al BI-op-se): See BIOPSY.

FROZEN SECTION (fro-zen SEK-shun): The quick preparation of a biopsy sample for examination during an actual surgical procedure. Tissue is taken from the operating room to the pathology laboratory and frozen. It is then thinly sliced and immediately examined under a microscope to determine if the sample is benign or malignant and to determine the status of margins.

GASTROSCOPY (gas-TROS-ko-pe): The insertion of an endoscope through the esophagus into the stomach for visual examination and/or biopsy of the stomach. When the upper portion of the small intestine is also visualized, the procedure is called *EGD* or *esophagogastroduodenoscopy.*

HOLTER ECG RECORDING (HOL-ter ECG re-KOR-ding): The electrocardiographic record of heart activity over an extended period of time. The Holter monitor is worn by the patient as he/she performs normal daily activities. It detects and aids in management of heart rhythm abnormalities. Also called *Holter monitoring.*

HYSTEROSCOPY (his-ter-OS-ko-pe): The insertion of an endoscope into the uterus for visual examination.

INCISIONAL BIOPSY (in-SIZ-in-al BI-op-se): See BIOPSY.

LAPAROSCOPY (lah-pah-ROS-ko-pe): The insertion of an endoscope into the abdomen. After the patient receives a local anesthetic, a laparoscope is inserted through an incision in the abdominal wall. This procedure affords the doctor a view of the abdominal cavity, the surface of the liver and spleen, and the pelvic region. The laparoscope is often used to perform fallopian tube ligation as a means of preventing pregnancy.

LARYNGOSCOPY (lah-rin-GOS-ko-pe): The insertion of an endoscope into the airway in order to visually examine the voice box (larynx). A laryngoscope transmits a magnified image of the larynx through a system of lenses and mirrors. The procedure can reveal tumors and explain changes in the voice. Sputum samples and tissue biopsies are obtained by using brushes or forceps attached to the laryngoscope.

MEDIASTINOSCOPY (me-de-ah-sti-NOS-ko-pe): The insertion of an endoscope into the mediastinum (the potential space in the chest between the lungs and in front of the heart). A mediastinoscope is inserted through a small incision in the neck while the patient is under anesthesia. This procedure is used to biopsy lymph nodes and to examine other structures within the mediastinum.

NEEDLE BIOPSY (NE-dl BI-op-se): See BIOPSY.

OTOSCOPIC EXAMINATION (o-to-SKOP-ic eks-am-ih-NA-shun): A physician uses an otoscope inserted into the ear canal to check for obstructions (e.g., wax), infection, fluid, and eardrum perforations or scarring.

OPHTHALMOSCOPIC EXAMINATION (of-thal-mo-SKOP-ic eks-am-ih-NA-shun): A physician uses an ophthalmoscope to look directly into the eye, evaluating the lens for cataracts, and the optic nerve, retina, and blood vessels in the back of the eye.

PALPATION (pal-PA-shun): Examination by touch. This is a technique of manual physical examination by which a doctor feels underlying tissues and organs through the skin.

PAP SMEAR (pap smer): The insertion of a cotton swab or wooden spatula into the vagina to obtain a sample of cells from the outer surface of the cervix (neck of the uterus). The cells are then smeared on a glass slide, preserved, and sent to the laboratory for microscopic examination. This test for cervical cancer was developed and named after the late Dr. George Papanicolaou. Results are reported as a Grade I–IV (I = normal, II = inflammatory, III = suspicious of malignancy, IV = malignancy).

PARACENTESIS (pah-rah-sen-TE-sis): Surgical puncture of the membrane surrounding the abdomen (peritoneum) to remove fluid from the abdominal cavity. Fluid is drained for analysis and to prevent its accumulation in the abdomen. Also known as *abdominocentesis*.

PELVIC EXAMINATION (PEL-vik eks-am-ih-NA-shun): Physician examines female sex organs and checks the uterus and ovaries for enlargement, cysts, tumors, or abnormal bleeding. This is also known as an "internal exam."

PERCUSSION (per-KUSH-un): The technique of striking a part of the body with short, sharp taps of the fingers to determine the size, density, and position of the underlying parts by the sound obtained. Percussion is commonly used on the abdomen to examine the liver.

PROCTOSIGMOIDOSCOPY (prok-to-sig-moy-DOS-ko-pe): The insertion of an endoscope through the anus to examine the first 10 to 12 inches of the rectum and colon. When the sigmoid colon is visualized using a longer endoscope, the procedure is called *sigmoidoscopy*. The procedure detects polyps, malignant tumors, and sources of bleeding.

PULMONARY FUNCTION STUDY (PUL-mon-nah-re FUNG-shun STUH-de): The measurement of the air taken into and exhaled from the lungs by means of an instrument called a *spirometer*. The test may be abnormal in patients with asthma, chronic bronchitis, emphysema, and occupational exposures to asbestos, chemicals, and dusts.

SIGMOIDOSCOPY (sig-moy-DOS-ko-pe): See PROCTOSIGMOIDOSCOPY.

STRESS TEST: This is an electrocardiogram taken during exercise. It may reveal hidden heart disease or confirm the cause of cardiac symptoms.

THORACENTESIS (thor-ah-sen-TE-sis): The insertion of a needle into the chest to remove fluid from the space surrounding the lungs (pleural cavity). After injection of a local anesthetic, a hollow needle is placed through the skin and muscles of the back and into the space between the lungs and chest wall. Fluid is then withdrawn by applying suction. Excess fluid *(pleural effusion)* may be a sign of infection or malignancy. This procedure is used for diagnostic studies, to drain a pleural effusion, or to re-expand a collapsed lung *(atelectasis)*.

THORACOSCOPY (tho-rah-KOS-ko-pe): The insertion of an endoscope through an incision in the chest in order to visually examine the surface of the lungs.

Laboratory Tests

The following laboratory tests are performed on samples of a patient's blood, *plasma* (fluid portion of the blood), *serum* (plasma minus clotting proteins and produced after blood has clotted), urine, feces, *sputum* (mucus coughed up from the lungs), *cerebrospinal fluid* (fluid within the spaces around the spinal cord and brain), and skin.

Pronunciation of each term is given with its meaning. The syllable that gets the accent is in CAPITAL LETTERS. Terms in SMALL CAPITAL LETTERS are defined elsewhere in the appendix.

ACID PHOSPHATASE (AH-sid FOS-fah-tas): Measures the amount of an enzyme called *acid phosphatase* in serum. Enzyme levels are elevated in metastatic prostate cancer. Moderate elevations of this enzyme occur in diseases of bone and when breast cancer cells invade bone tissue.

ALBUMIN (al-BU-min): Measures *albumin* (protein) in both serum and in urine. A decrease of albumin in serum indicates disease of the kidneys, malnutrition, or liver disease or may occur in extensive loss of protein in the gut or from the skin, as in a burn. The presence of albumin in the urine *(albuminuria)* indicates malfunction of the kidney.

ALKALINE PHOSPHATASE (AL-kah-lin FOS-fah-tas): Measures the amount of *alkaline phosphatase* (an enzyme found on cell membranes) in serum. Levels are elevated in liver diseases (such as hepatitis and hepatoma), and in bone disease and bone cancer. The laboratory symbol is *alk phos.*

ALPHA-FETOPROTEIN (al-fa-fe-to-PRO-ten): Test for the presence of a protein called alpha-globulin in serum. The protein is normally present in the serum of the fetus, infant, and pregnant women. In fetuses with abnormalities of the brain and spinal cord, the protein leaks into the amniotic fluid surrounding the fetus and is an indicator of spinal tube defect (spina bifida) or anencephaly (lack of brain development). High levels are found in patients with cancer of the liver and other malignancies (testicular and ovarian cancers). Serum levels monitor the effectiveness of cancer treatment. Elevated levels are also seen in benign liver disease such as cirrhosis and viral hepatitis. The laboratory symbol is *AFP.*

ANA: See ANTINUCLEAR ANTIBODY TEST.

ANTINUCLEAR ANTIBODY TEST (an-tih-NU-kle-ar AN-tih-bod-e test):   A sample of plasma is tested for the presence of antibodies that are found in patients with systemic lupus erythematosus. Laboratory symbol is *ANA*.

BENCE JONES PROTEIN (BENS jonz PRO-ten): Measures the presence of the Bence Jones protein in serum or urine. Bence Jones protein is a fragment of a normal serum protein, an immunoglobulin, produced by cancerous bone marrow cells (myeloma cells). Normally it is not found in either blood or urine, but in *multiple myeloma* (a malignant condition of bone marrow) high levels of Bence Jones protein are detected in urine and serum.

BILIRUBIN (bil-eh-RU-bin):   Measures the amount of *bilirubin,* an orange-brown pigment, in serum and urine. Bilirubin is derived from hemoglobin, the oxygen-carrying protein in red blood cells. Its presence in high concentration in serum and urine causes jaundice (yellow coloration of the skin) and may indicate disease of the liver, obstruction of bile ducts, or a type of anemia that leads to excessive destruction of red blood cells.

BLOOD CHEMISTRY PROFILE: This comprehensive blood test provides information regarding the function of several body systems. Tests include calcium (bones), phosphorus (bones), urea (kidney), creatinine (kidney), bilirubin (liver), SGOT (liver and heart muscle) and SGPT (liver), alkaline phosphatase (liver and bone), globulin (liver and immune disorders), and albumin (liver and kidney). Laboratory symbol is *SMAC*.

BLOOD CULTURE (blud KUL-chur):   To test for infection in the bloodstream, a sample of blood is added to a special medium (food) that promotes the growth of microorganisms. The medium is then examined by a medical technologist for evidence of bacteria or other microbes.

BLOOD UREA NITROGEN (blud u-RE-ah NI-tro-jen): Measures the amount of urea (nitrogen-containing waste material) in serum. A high level of serum urea indicates poor kidney function, since it is the kidney's job to remove urea from the bloodstream and filter it into urine. Laboratory symbol is *BUN*.

CALCIUM (KAL-se-um): Measures the amount of calcium in serum, plasma, or whole blood. Low blood levels are associated with abnormal functioning of nerves and muscles, and high blood levels indicate loss of calcium from bones, excessive intake of calcium, disease of the parathyroid glands, or cancer. Laboratory symbol is *Ca*.

CARBON DIOXIDE (KAR-bon di-OK-side): This gas, produced in tissues and eliminated by the lungs, is measured in the blood. Abnormal levels may reflect lung disorders. Laboratory symbol is CO_2.

CARCINOEMBRYONIC ANTIGEN (kar-sih-no-em-bree-ON-ik AN-ti-jen): A plasma test for a protein normally found in the blood of human fetuses and produced in healthy adults only in a very small amount, if at all. High levels of this antigen may be a sign of one of a variety of cancers, especially colon or pancreatic cancer. This test is used to monitor the response of patients to cancer treatment. Laboratory abbreviation is *CEA*.

CEREBROSPINAL FLUID (seh-re-bro-SPI-nal FLU-id): Chemical tests are performed on specimens of cerebrospinal fluid removed by *lumbar puncture*. The fluid is tested for protein, sugar, and blood cells. It is also cultured to detect microorganisms. Abnormal conditions such as meningitis, brain tumor, and encephalitis are detected using this test. Laboratory abbreviation is *CSF*.

CHOLESTEROL (ko-LES-ter-ol): Measures the amount of cholesterol (substance found in animal fats and oils, egg yolks, and milk) in serum or plasma. Normal values vary for age and diet; levels above 200 mg/dl indicate a need for further testing and efforts to reduce cholesterol level, since high levels are associated with hardening of arteries and heart disease. Blood is also tested for the presence of a lipoprotein substance that is a combination of cholesterol and protein. High levels of *HDL* (high-density lipoprotein) cholesterol in the blood are beneficial, since HDL cholesterol promotes the removal and excretion of excess cholesterol from the body, while high levels of low-density lipoprotein *(LDL)* are dangerous.

COMPLETE BLOOD COUNT: Numbers of leukocytes (white blood cells), erythrocytes (red blood cells), and platelets (clotting cells) are determined. The CBC is useful in diagnosing anemia, infection, and blood cell disorders, such as leukemia.

CREATINE KINASE (KRE-ah-tin KI-nas): Serum test to detect levels of creatine kinase, a blood enzyme. Creatine kinase is normally found in heart muscle, brain tissue, and skeletal muscle. The presence of one form *(isoenzyme)* of creatine kinase (either CK-MB or CK2) in the blood is strongly indicative of recent myocardial infarction (heart attack), since the enzyme is released from heart muscle when the muscle is damaged or dying.

CREATININE (kre-AT-tih-nin): Measures the amount of creatinine, a nitrogen-containing waste material, in serum or plasma. It is the most reliable test for kidney function. Since creatinine is normally produced as a protein breakdown product in muscle and excreted by the kidney in urine, an elevation in the creatinine level in the blood indicates a disturbance of kidney function. Elevations are also seen in high protein diets and dehydration.

CREATININE CLEARANCE (kre-AT-ih-nin KLER-ans): Measures the rate at which creatinine is cleared (filtered) by the kidneys from the blood. If creatinine clearance is low, it indicates that the kidneys are not functioning effectively to clear creatinine from the bloodstream and filter it into urine.

CULTURE (KUL-chur): This test identifies microorganisms in a special laboratory medium (fluid, solid, or semisolid material). In *sensitivity* tests, culture plates containing a specific microorganism are prepared, and antibiotic-containing discs are applied to the culture surface. Following overnight incubation, the area surrounding the disc (where growth was inhibited) is measured to determine if the antibiotic is effective against the specific organism.

DIFFERENTIAL (di-fer-EN-shul): See WHITE BLOOD CELL COUNT.

ELECTROLYTES (e-LEK-tro-litz): Tests on serum or whole blood to determine the concentration of *electrolytes* (chemical substances which are capable of conducting an electric current). When dissolved in water, electrolytes break apart into charged particles *(ions)*. Positively charged electrolytes are *sodium* (Na^+), *potassium* (K^+), *calcium* (CA^{++}), and *magnesium* (MG^{++}). Negatively charged electrolytes are *chloride* (Cl^-) and *bicarbonate* (HCO_3^-). These charged particles should be present at all times for proper functioning of cells. An electrolyte imbalance occurs when serum concentration is either too high or too low. Calcium imbalance can affect the bones, kidneys, gastrointestinal tract, and neuromuscular activity, while sodium affects blood pressure, nerve functioning, and fluid levels surrounding cells. Potassium affects heart and muscular activity.

ELECTROPHORESIS: See SERUM PROTEIN ELECTROPHORESIS.

ELISA (eh-LI-zah): A laboratory assay (test) for the presence of antibodies to the AIDS virus. If a patient tests positive, it is likely that his/her blood contains the AIDS virus (HIV or human immunodeficiency virus). The presence of the virus stimulates white blood cells to make antibodies that are detected by the ELISA assay. This is the first test done to detect AIDS infection and is followed by a *Western blot* test to confirm the results. ELISA is an acronym for *e*nzyme-*l*inked *i*mmuno*s*orbent *as*-say.

ERYTHROCYTE SEDIMENTATION RATE (eh-RITH-ro-sit sed-ih-men-TA-shun rat): Measures the rate at which red blood cells (erythrocytes) in well-mixed venous blood settle to the bottom (sediment) of a test tube. If the rate of sedimentation is markedly slow (elevated sed rate), it may indicate inflammatory conditions, such as rheumatoid arthritis, or conditions that produce excessive proteins in the blood. Laboratory symbols are *ESR* and *sed rate.*

ESTRADIOL (es-tra-DI-ol): A test for the concentration of estradiol, which is a form of estrogen (female hormone) in serum, plasma, or urine.

ESTROGEN RECEPTOR ASSAY (ES-tro-jen rih-SEP-ter As-a): This test, performed at the time of a biopsy, determines if a sample of tumor contains an estrogen receptor protein. The protein, if present on breast cancer cells, combines with estrogen, allowing estrogen to promote the growth of the tumor. Thus, if an estrogen receptor assay test is positive (the protein is present) then treatment with an anti-estrogen drug would retard tumor growth. If the assay is negative (the protein is not present), then the tumor would not be affected by anti-estrogen drug treatment.

GLOBULIN (GLOB-u-lin): Measured in serum, *globulins* are proteins that bind to and destroy foreign substances (antigens). Globulins are made by cells of the immune system. Gamma globulin is one type of globulin that contains antibodies to fight disease.

GLUCOSE (GLU-kos): Measures the amount of glucose (sugar) in serum and plasma. High levels of glucose *(hyperglycemia)* indicate diseases such as diabetes mellitus and hyperthyroidism. Glucose is also measured in urine, and its presence indicates diabetes mellitus.

GLUCOSE TOLERANCE TEST (GLU-kos TOL-er-ans test): In the first part of this test, blood and urine samples are taken after the patient has fasted. Then, a solution of glucose is given by mouth. One-half hour after the glucose is taken, blood and urine samples are obtained again, and are collected every hour for 4 to 5 hours. The test determines how the body uses glucose and can indicate abnormal conditions such as diabetes mellitus, hypoglycemia, and liver or adrenal gland dysfunction.

HEMATOCRIT (he-MAT-o-krit): Measures the percentage of red blood cells in the blood. The normal range is 40 to 50 per cent in males and 37 to 47 per cent in females. A low hematocrit indicates anemia. Laboratory symbol is *Hct*.

HEMOGLOBIN ASSAY (HE-mo-glo-bin AS-a): Measures the concentration of hemoglobin in blood. The normal blood hemoglobin ranges are 13.5 to 18.0 gm/dl in adult males and 12.0 to 16.0 gm/dl in adult females. Laboratory symbol is *Hgb*.

HEMOCCULT TEST (he-mo-KULT test): A small sample of stool is tested for otherwise inapparent ("occult" means "hidden") traces of blood. The sample is placed on the surface of a collection kit and reacts with a chemical (e.g., guaiac). A positive result may indicate bleeding from polyps, ulcers, or malignant tumors.

HUMAN CHORIONIC GONADOTROPIN (HU-man kor-e-ON-ik go-nad-o-TRO-pin): Measures the concentration of human chorionic gonadotropin (a hormone secreted by cells of the fetal placenta) in urine. It is detected in urine within days after fertilization of egg and sperm cells and provides the basis of the most commonly used pregnancy test. Laboratory symbol is *hCG*.

IMMUNOASSAY (im-u-no-AS-a): A method of testing blood and urine for the concentration of various chemicals, such as hormones, drugs, or proteins. The technique makes use of the immunological reaction between antigens and antibodies. An *assay* is a determination of the amount of any particular substance in a mixture.

PKU TEST: This test determines if the urine of a newborn baby contains substances called *phenylketones*. If so, the condition is called *phenylketonuria (PKU)*. Phenylketonuria occurs in infants born lacking a specific enzyme. If the enzyme is missing, high levels of *phenylalanine* (an amino acid) accumulate in the blood, affecting the infant's brain and causing mental retardation. This situation is prevented by placing the infant on a special diet that prevents accumulation of phenylalanine in the bloodstream.

PLATELET COUNT (PLAT-let kownt):   Determines the number of clotting cells (platelets) in a sample of blood.

POTASSIUM (po-TAHS-e-um):   Measures the concentration of potassium in serum. Potassium combines with other minerals (such as calcium) and is an important chemical for proper functioning of muscles, especially the heart muscle. Laboratory symbol is K^+. See also ELECTROLYTES.

PROGESTERONE RECEPTOR ASSAY (pro-JES-ter-on rih-SEP-ter AS-a):   This test determines if a sample of tumor contains a progesterone receptor protein. If positive, it identifies a tumor that would be responsive to antiprogesterone hormone therapy.

PROSTATE-SPECIFIC ANTIGEN (pros-TAT spe-SI-fic AN-ti-jen):   This blood test measures the amount of an antigen that is elevated in all patients with prostatic cancer and in some with an inflamed prostate gland. Laboratory symbol is *PSA*.

PROTEIN ELECTROPHORESIS: See SERUM PROTEIN ELECTROPHORESIS.

PROTHROMBIN TIME (pro-THROM-bin tim):   Measures the activity of factors in the blood that participate in clotting. Deficiency of any of these factors can lead to a prolonged prothrombin time and difficulty in blood clotting. The test is important as a monitor for patients who are taking anticoagulants, substances that block the activity of blood clotting factors, and increase the risk of bleeding.

PSA: See PROSTATE-SPECIFIC ANTIGEN.

RED BLOOD CELL COUNT: This test counts the number of erythrocytes in a sample of blood. A low red blood cell count may indicate anemia. A high RBC count can indicate *polycythemia vera.*

RHEUMATOID FACTOR (RU-mah-toyd FAK-tor): Detects an abnormal protein *(rheumatoid factor)* present in the serum of patients with rheumatoid arthritis.

SERUM GLUTAMIC-OXALOACETIC TRANSAMINASE (SE-rum glu-TAM-ik oks-al-ah-SE-tik trans-AM-in-as): Measures the amount of the enzyme *glutamate-oxaloacetate transaminase (aspartate transaminase)* in serum. The enzyme is normally present, but when there is damage to heart (heart attack) or liver cells, it is released by the damaged tissue and accumulates in the blood. Laboratory symbol is *SGOT* or *AST.*

SERUM GLUTAMIC-PYRUVIC TRANSAMINASE (SE-rum glu-TAM-ic pi-RU-vik trans-AM-in-as): Measures the amount of the enzyme *glutamate-pyruvic transaminase (alanine transaminase)* in serum. The enzyme is normally in the blood but accumulates in abnormally high amounts when there is acute damage to liver cells as in hepatitis, infectious mononucleosis, and obstructive jaundice. Laboratory symbol is *SGPT* or *ALT.*

SERUM PROTEIN ELECTROPHORESIS (SE-rum PRO-ten e-lek-tro-for-E-sis): This procedure separates proteins using an electric current. The material tested, such as serum, containing various proteins, is placed on paper or gel or in liquid and, under the influence of an electric current, the proteins separate (-phoresis means separation) so that they can be identified and measured. The procedure is also known as *protein electrophoresis.*

SGOT: See SERUM GLUTAMIC-OXALOACETIC TRANSAMINASE.

SGPT: See SERUM GLUTAMIC-PYRUVIC TRANSAMINASE.

SKIN TESTS: In these tests, substances are applied to the skin or injected under the skin, and the reaction of immune cells in the skin is observed. These tests detect a person's sensitivity to substances such as dust or pollen. They can also indicate if a person has been exposed to the bacteria that cause tuberculosis or diphtheria.

SODIUM: See ELECTROLYTES.

SMAC: See BLOOD CHEMISTRY PROFILE.

SPUTUM TEST (SPU-tum test):   Examines mucus that is coughed up from a patient's lungs. The sputum is examined microscopically and chemically, and cultured for the presence of microorganisms.

THYROID FUNCTION TESTS (THI-royd FUNK-shun tests):   These tests measure the levels of thyroid hormones, such as *thyroxine* (T_4) and *triiodothyronine* (T_3) in serum. *Thyroid-stimulating hormone (TSH),* which is produced by the pituitary gland and stimulates the release of T_4 and T_3 from the thyroid gland, can also be measured in serum. These tests aid in the diagnosis of hypo- and hyperthyroidism and are helpful in monitoring response to thyroid treatment.

TRIGLYCERIDES (tri-GLIS-er-idz):   Determines the amount of *triglycerides* (fats) in the serum. Elevated triglycerides are considered an important risk factor for the development of heart disease.

URIC ACID (UR-ik AS-id):   Measures the amount of *uric acid* (a nitrogen-containing waste material) in the serum and urine. High serum levels indicate a type of arthritis called *gout.* In gout, uric acid accumulates as crystals in joints and in tissues. High levels of uric acid may also cause kidney stones.

URINALYSIS (u-rih-NAL-ih-sis):   Examination of urine as an aid in the diagnosis of disease. Routine urinalysis involves observation of unusual color or odor; determining specific gravity (amount of materials dissolved in urine); chemical tests (for protein, sugar, acetone); and microscopic examination for bacteria, blood cells, and sediment. Urinalysis is used to detect abnormal functioning of the kidneys and bladder, infections, abnormal growths, and diabetes mellitus. Laboratory symbol is *UA*.

WESTERN BLOT (WES-tern blot): This test is more specific than the ELISA to detect infection by *HIV* (AIDS virus). A patient's serum is mixed with purified proteins from HIV and the reaction is examined. If the patient has made antibodies to HIV, those antibodies will react with the purified HIV proteins, and the test will be positive.

WHITE BLOOD CELL (WBC) COUNT: Determines the number of leukocytes in the blood. Higher than normal counts can indicate the presence of infection or leukemia. A *differential* is the percentages of different types of white blood cells (neutrophils, eosinophils, basophils, lymphocytes, and monocytes) in a sample of blood. It gives more specific information about leukocytes and aids in diagnosis of allergic diseases, disorders of the immune system, and various forms of leukemia.

PART II

USEFUL INFORMATION

Acronyms for Selected Health Care Organizations, Associations, and Agencies*

AAAA	American Academy of Anesthesiologist's Assistants
AAATP	Association for Anesthesiologist's Assistants Training Program
AAB	American Association of Bioanalysts
AABB	American Association of Blood Banks
AACA	American Association of Clinical Anatomists
AACAHPO	American Association of Certified Allied Health Personnel in Ophthalmology
AACC	American Association for Clinical Chemistry
AACCN	American Association of Critical Care Nurses
AACN	American Association of Colleges of Nursing
AADS	American Association of Dental Schools
AAFP	American Academy of Family Physicians
AAHA	American Academy of Health Administration

Chart continued on following page

* From O'Toole, M: Miller-Keane Encyclopedia & Dictionary Of Medicine, Nursing & Allied Health, 6th ed. Philadelphia, W.B. Saunders, 1997.

Acronyms for Selected Health Care Organizations, Associations, and Agencies
Continued

AAHC	Association of Academic Health Centers
AAHE	Association for the Advancement of Health Education
AAHP	American Association of Hospital Planners
AAHPER	American Association for Health, Physical Education, and Recreation
AAMA	American Association of Medical Assistants
AAMC	Association of American Medical Colleges
AAMI	Association for the Advancement of Medical Instrumentation
AAMT	American Association for Medical Transcription
AAN	American Academy of Neurology
AANA	American Association of Nurse Anesthetists
AAO	American Association of Ophthalmology
AAO	American Association of Orthodontists
AAOHN	American Association of Occupational Health Nurses
AAP	American Academy of Pediatrics
AAPA	American Academy of Physicians Assistants
AAPMR	American Academy of Physical Medicine and Rehabilitation
AARC	American Association for Respiratory Care
AART	American Association for Rehabilitation Therapy
AATA	American Art Therapy Association
AATS	American Association for Thoracic Surgery

Acronyms for Selected Health Care
Organizations, Associations, and Agencies
Continued

ABCP	American Board of Cardiovascular Perfusion
ABNFHE	Association of Black Nursing Faculty in Higher Education
ACC	American College of Cardiology
ACCP	American College of Chest Physicians
ACEN	Academy of Chief Executive Nurses (Canada)
ACEP	American College of Emergency Physicians
ACHA	American College of Hospital Administrators
ACNM	American College of Nurse-Midwives
ACP	American College of Physicians
ACR	American College of Radiology
ACS	American College of Surgeons
ACTA	American Cardiovascular Technologists Association
ACTA	American Corrective Therapy Association
ADA	American Dental Association
ADA	American Dietetic Association
ADAA	American Dental Assistants Association
ADHA	American Dental Hygienists' Association
ADTA	American Dance Therapy Association
AES	American Electroencephalographic Society
AHA	American Hospital Association
AHIMA	American Health Information Management Association
AHPA	American Health Planning Association

Chart continued on following page

Acronyms for Selected Health Care Organizations, Associations, and Agencies
Continued

AIBS	American Institute of Biological Sciences
AIHA	American Industrial Hygiene Association
AIUM	American Institute of Ultrasound in Medicine
AMA	American Medical Association
AMEA	American Medical Electroencephalographic Association
AMI	Association of Medical Illustrators
AmSECT	American Society of Extra-Corporeal Technology
AMT	American Medical Technologists
ANA	American Nurses Association
ANF	American Nurses Foundation
ANNA	American Nephrology Nurses' Association
ANRC	American National Red Cross
AOA	American Optometric Association
AOA	American Osteopathic Association
AONE	American Organization of Nurse Executives
AORN	Association of Operating Room Nurses
AOTA	American Occupational Therapy Association
APA	American Podiatry Association
APA	American Psychiatric Association
APA	American Psychological Association
APAP	Association of Physician Assistants Programs
APHA	American Public Health Association
APIC	Association of Practitioners in Infection Control
APTA	American Physical Therapy Association

Acronyms for Selected Health Care
Organizations, Associations, and Agencies
Continued

ARCA	American Rehabilitation Counseling Association
ARN	Association of Rehabilitation Nurses
ASA	American Society of Anesthesiologists
ASAHP	American Society of Allied Health Professionals
ASC	American Society of Cytotechnology
ASCP	American Society of Clinical Pathologists
ASE	American Society of Echocardiography
ASET	American Society of Electroencephalographic Technologists
ASHA	American Speech and Hearing Association
ASIA	American Spinal Injury Association
ASIM	American Society of Internal Medicine
ASM	American Society of Microbiology
ASMT	American Society for Medical Technology
ASNSA	American Society of Nursing Service Administrators
ASPAN	American Society of Post Anesthesia Nurses
ASPH	Association of Schools of Public Health
ASRT	American Society of Radiologic Technologists
AST	Association of Surgical Technologists
ASUTS	American Society of Ultrasound Technical Specialists
ATS	American Thoracic Society

Chart continued on following page

Acronyms for Selected Health Care
Organizations, Associations, and Agencies
Continued

AUPHA	Association of University Programs in Health Administration
AVA	American Vocational Association
AVMA	American Veterinary Medical Association
CAP	College of American Pathologists
CAHEA (AMA)	Committee on Allied Health Education and Accreditation of the American Medical Association
CCHFA	Canadian Council of Health Facilities Accreditation
CCHSE	Canadian Council of Health Service Executives
CDC	Centers for Disease Control and Prevention
CGFNS	Commission on Graduates of Foreign Nursing Schools
CGNA	Canadian Gerontological Nursing Association
CME (AMA)	Council on Medical Education of the American Medical Association
CNA	Canadian Nurses Association
COEAMRA	Council on Education of the American Medical Record Association
DHHS	Department of Health and Human Services
ENA	Emergency Nurses Association
FDA	Food and Drug Administration
HCFA	Health Care Financing Administration
HRA	Health Resources Administration
HSCA	Health Sciences Communications Association
HSRA	Health Services and Resources Administration

Acronyms for Selected Health Care Organizations, Associations, and Agencies
Continued

IAET	International Association for Enterostomal Therapy
ISCV	International Society for Cardiovascular Surgery
JCAHO	Joint Commission on the Accreditation of Healthcare Organizations
JCAHPO	Joint Commission on Allied Health Personnel in Ophthalmology
MLA	Medical Library Association
MTIA	Medical Transcription Industry Alliance
NAACLS	National Accrediting Agency for Clinical Laboratory Science
NAACOG	Nurses Association of the American College of Obstetrics and Gynecology
NACA	National Advisory Council on Aging—Canadian
NACT	National Alliance of Cardiovascular Technologists
NADONA/LTC	National Association of Directors of Nursing Administration in Long Term Care
NAEMT	National Association of Emergency Medical Technicians
NAHC	National Association of Home Care
NAHSR	National Association of Human Services Technologists
NAMH	National Association of Mental Health
NAMT	National Association for Music Therapy
NANDA	North American Nursing Diagnosis Association

Chart continued on following page

Acronyms for Selected Health Care
Organizations, Associations, and Agencies
Continued

NANPRH	National Association of Nurse Practitioners in Reproductive Health
NANT	National Association of Nephrology Technologists
NAPNES	National Association for Practical Nurse Education and Services
NARF	National Association of Rehabilitation Facilities
NASW	National Association of Social Workers
NATTS	National Association of Trade and Technical Schools
NCEHPHP	National Council on the Education of Health Professionals in Health Promotion
NCRE	National Council on Rehabilitation Education
NEHA	National Environmental Health Association
NFLPN	National Federation of Licensed Practical Nurses
NHC	National Health Council
NIH	National Institutes of Health
NIOSH	National Institute of Occupational Safety and Health
NKF	National Kidney Foundation
NLN	National League for Nursing
NNBA	National Nurses in Business Association
NRCA	National Rehabilitation Counseling Association
NREMT	National Registry of Emergency Medical Technicians
NSCPT	National Society for Cardiopulmonary Technology

Acronyms for Selected Health Care Organizations, Associations, and Agencies
Continued

NSH	National Society for Histotechnology
NSNA	National Student Nurses Association
NTRS	National Therapeutic Recreation Society
OAA	Opticians Association of America
ONS	Oncology Nurses Association
SAAABB	Subcommittee on Accreditation of the American Association of Blood Banks
SDMS	Society of Diagnostic Medical Sonographers
SNIVT	Society of Non-Invasive Vascular Technology
SNM	Society of Nuclear Medicine
SNM-TS	Society of Nuclear Medicine—Technologists Section
SPHE	Society of Public Health Educators
STS	Society of Thoracic Surgeons
SVS	Society for Vascular Surgery
TAANA	American Association of Nurse Attorneys
USPHS	United States Public Health Service
VA	Veterans Affairs
WHO	World Health Organization

Professional Designations for Health Care Providers*

Degrees, certifications, memberships and other initials that precede or follow the names of health care providers often provide helpful information regarding their area of expertise and level of practice. The following list identifies commonly used designations in English speaking countries, particularly the United States and Canada.

ANP	Adult Nurse Practitioner
ARNP	Advanced Registered Nurse Practitioner
BA	Bachelor of Arts
BB(ASCP)	Technologist in Blood Banking certified by The American Society of Clinical Pathologists
BDentSci	Bachelor of Dental Science
BDS	Bachelor of Dental Surgery
BDSc	Bachelor of Dental Science
BHS	Bachelor of Health Science
BHyg	Bachelor of Hygiene
BM	Bachelor of Medicine
BMed	Bachelor of Medicine
BMedBiol	Bachelor of Medical Biology
BMedSci	Bachelor of Medical Science
BMic	Bachelor of Microbiology
BMS	Bachelor of Medical Science
BMT	Bachelor of Medical Technology

Chart continued on following page

---

*From O'Toole M: Miller-Keane Encyclopedia & Dictionary Of Medicine, Nursing & Allied Health, 6th ed. Philadelphia, W.B. Saunders, 1997.

Professional Designations for Health Care Providers *Continued*

BO	Bachelor of Osteopathy
BP	Bachelor of Pharmacy
BPH	Bachelor of Public Health
BPharm	Bachelor of Pharmacy
BPHEng	Bachelor of Public Health Engineering
BPHN	Bachelor of Public Health Nursing
BPsTh	Bachelor of Psychotherapy
BS	Bachelor of Science
BSM	Bachelor of Science in Medicine
BSN	Bachelor of Science in Nursing
BSPh	Bachelor of Science in Pharmacy
BSS	Bachelor of Sanitary Science
BVMS	Bachelor of Veterinary Medicine and Science
BVSc	Bachelor of Veterinary Science
CALN	Clinical Administrative Liaison Nurse
C(ASCP)	Technologist in Chemistry certified by the American Society of Clinical Pathologists
CB	Bachelor of Surgery
CCRN	Critical Care Registered Nurse
CDA	Certified Dental Assistant
CEN	Certificate for Emergency Nursing
CEO	Chief Executive Officer
ChB	Bachelor of Surgery
CHCRM	Certified Health Care Risk Manager
ChD	Doctor of Surgery
ChM	Master of Surgery
CIH	Certificate in Industrial Health
CLA	Certified Laboratory Assistant
CLS	Clinical Laboratory Scientist
CLS(NCA)	Clinical Laboratory Scientist certified by the National Certification Agency for Medical Laboratory Personnel
CLT	Certified Laboratory Technician; Clinical Laboratory Technician

Professional Designations for Health Care Providers *Continued*

CLT(NCA)	Laboratory Technician certified by the National Certification Agency for Medical Laboratory Personnel
CM	Master of Surgery
CMA	Certified Medical Assistant
CMO	Chief Medical Officer
CMT	Certified Medical Transcriptionist
CNM	Certified Nurse Midwife
CNMT	Certified Nuclear Medicine Technologist
CNP	Community Nurse Practitioner
CNS	Clinical Nurse Specialist
CORN	Certified Operating Room Nurse
COTA	Certified Occupational Therapy Assistant
CPAN	Certified Post Anesthesia Nurse
CPH	Certificate in Public Health
CPNP	Certified Pediatric Nurse Practitioner
CRNA	Certified Registered Nurse Anesthetist
CRRN	Certified Registered Rehabilitation Nurse
CRTT	Certified Respiratory Therapy Technician
CT(ASCP)	Cytotechnologist certified by the American Society of Clinical Pathologists
CTR	Certified Tumor Registrar
CURN	Certified Urological Registered Nurse
CVO	Chief Veterinary Officer
DA	Dental Assistant; Diploma in Anesthetics
DC	Doctor of Chiropractic
DCH	Diploma in Child Health
DCh	Doctor of Surgery
DChO	Doctor of Ophthalmic Surgery
DCM	Doctor of Comparative Medicine
DCOG	Diploma of the College of Obstetricians and Gynaecologists

Chart continued on following page

Professional Designations for Health Care Providers *Continued*

DCP	Diploma in Clinical Pathology; Diploma in Clinical Psychology
DDH	Diploma in Dental Health
DDM	Doctor of Dental Medicine; Diploma in Dermatologic Medicine
DDO	Diploma in Dental Orthopaedics
DDR	Diploma in Diagnostic Radiology
DDS	Doctor of Dental Surgery
DDSc	Doctor of Dental Science
DFHom	Diploma of the Faculty of Homeopathy
DHg	Doctor of Hygiene
DHy	Doctor of Hygiene
DHyg	Doctor of Hygiene
Dip	Diplomate
DipBact	Diploma in Bacteriology
DipChem	Diploma in Chemistry
DipClinPath	Diploma in Clinical Pathology
DipMicrobiol	Diploma in Microbiology
DipSocMed	Diploma in Social Medicine
DLM(ASCP)	Diplomate in Laboratory Management certified by the American Society of Clinical Pathologists
DMD	Doctor of Dental Medicine
DMT	Doctor of Medical Technology
DMV	Doctor of Veterinary Medicine
DN	Doctor of Nursing
DNE	Doctor of Nursing Education
DNS	Doctor of Nursing Science
DNSc	Doctor of Nursing Science
DO	Doctor of Osteopathy; Doctor of Optometry; Doctor of Ophthalmology
DON	Director of Nursing
DOS	Doctor of Ocular Science; Doctor of Optical Science
DP	Doctor of Pharmacy; Doctor of Podiatry
DPH	Doctor of Public Hygiene; Doctor of Public Health

Professional Designations for Health Care Providers *Continued*

DPhC	Doctor of Pharmaceutical Chemistry
DPHN	Doctor of Public Health Nursing
DPhys	Diploma in Physiotherapy
DPM	Doctor of Podiatric Medicine; Doctor of Physical Medicine; Doctor of Preventive Medicine; Doctor of Psychiatric Medicine
Dr	Doctor
DrHyg	Doctor of Hygiene
DrMed	Doctor of Medicine
DrPH	Doctor of Public Health; Doctor of Public Hygiene
DSc	Doctor of Science
DSE	Doctor of Sanitary Engineering
DSIM	Doctor of Science in Industrial Medicine
DSSc	Diploma in Sanitary Science
DVM	Doctor of Veterinary Medicine
DVMS	Doctor of Veterinary Medicine and Surgery
DVR	Doctor of Veterinary Radiology
DVS	Doctor of Veterinary Science; Doctor of Veterinary Medicine
DVSc	Doctor of Veterinary Science
Ed.D.	Doctor of Education
ET	Enterostomal Therapist
FAAN	Fellow of the American Academy of Nurses
FACA	Fellow of the American College of Anesthetists; Fellow of the American College of Angiology; Fellow of the American College of Apothecaries
FACAI	Fellow of the American College of Allergists
FACC	Fellow of the American College of Cardiologists
FACCP	Fellow of the American College of Chest Physicians

Chart continued on following page

Professional Designations for Health Care
Providers *Continued*

FACD	Fellow of the American College of Dentists
FACFP	Fellow of the American College of Family Physicians
FACG	Fellow of the American College of Gastroenterology
FACHA	Fellow of the American College of Health Administrators
FACOG	Fellow of the American College of Obstetricians and Gynecologists
FACP	Fellow of the American College of Physicians
FACPM	Fellow of the American College of Preventive Medicine
FACS	Fellow of the American College of Surgeons
FACSM	Fellow of the American College of Sports Medicine
FAMA	Fellow of the American Medicine Association
FAOTA	Fellow of the American Occupational Therapy Association
FAPA	Fellow of the American Psychiatric Association
FAPHA	Fellow of the American Public Health Association
FBPsS	Fellow of the British Psychological Association
FCAP	Fellow of the College of American Pathologists
FCMS	Fellow of the College of Medicine and Surgery
FCO	Fellow of the College of Osteopathy
FCPS	Fellow of the College of Physicians and Surgeons
FCSP	Fellow of the Chartered Society of Physiotherapy

Professional Designations for Health Care Providers *Continued*

FCST	Fellow of the College of Speech Therapists
FDS	Fellow in Dental Surgery
FDSRCSEng	Fellow in Dental Surgery of the Royal College of Surgeons of England
FFA	Fellow of the Faculty of Anesthetists
FFCM	Fellow of the Faculty of Community Medicine
FFD	Fellow in the Faculty of Dentistry
FFOM	Fellow of the Faculty of Occupational Medicine
FFR	Fellow of the Faculty of Radiologists
FIB	Fellow in the Institute of Biology
FICD	Fellow of the Institute of Canadian Dentists; Fellow of the International College of Dentists
FIMLT	Fellow of the Institute of Medical Laboratory Technology
FNP	Family Nurse Practitioner
FPS	Fellow of the Pathological Society
FRCD	Fellow of the Royal College of Dentists
FRCGP	Fellow of the Royal College of General Practitioners
FRCOG	Fellow of the Royal College of Obstetricians and Gynaecologists
FRCP	Fellow of the Royal College of Physicians
FRCPath	Fellow of the Royal College of Pathologists
FRCP(C)	Fellow of the Royal College of Physicians of Canada
FRCS	Fellow of the Royal College of Surgeons
FRCS(C)	Fellow of the Royal College of Surgeons of Canada

Chart continued on following page

GNP	Gerontological Nurse Practitioner
H(ASCP)	Technologist in Hematology certified by the American Society of Clinical Pathologists
HT(ASCP)	Histologic Technician certified by the American Society of Clinical Pathologists
HTL(ASCP)	Histotechnologist certified by the American Society of Clinical Pathologists
I(ASCP)	Technologist in Immunology certified by the American Society of Clinical Pathologists
LMCC	Licentiate of the Medical Council of Canada
LMRCP	Licentiate in Midwifery of the Royal College of Physicians
LPN	Licensed Practical Nurse
LVN	Licensed Vocational Nurse
MA	Master of Arts
M(ASCP)	Technologist in Microbiology certified by the American Society of Clinical Pathologists
MAT	Master of Arts in Teaching
MB	Bachelor of Medicine
MC	Mastery of Surgery
MCPS	Member of the College of Physicians and Surgeons
MD	Doctor of Medicine
MDentSc	Master of Dental Science
MDS	Master of Dental Surgery
MLT	Medical Laboratory Technician
MLT(ASCP)	Medical Laboratory Technician certified by the American Society of Clinical Pathologists
MMS	Master of Medical Science
MMSA	Master of Midwifery
MPH	Master of Public Health
MPharm	Master of Pharmacy

Professional Designations for Health Care
Providers *Continued*

MRad	Master of Radiology
MRL	Medical Records Librarian
MS	Master of Science; Master of Surgery
MSB	Master of Science in Bacteriology
MSc	Master of Science
MScD	Master of Dental Science
MScN	Master of Science in Nursing
MSN	Master of Science in Nursing
MSPH	Master of Science in Public Health
MSPhar	Master of Science in Pharmacy
MSSc	Master of Sanitary Science
MSW	Master of Social Work; Medical Social Worker
MT	Medical Technologist
MT(ASCP)	Medical Technologist certified by the American Society of Clinical Pathologists
MVD	Doctor of Veterinary Medicine
ND	Doctor of Nursing
NM(ASCP)	Technologist in Nuclear Medicine certified by the American Society of Clinical Pathologists
NP	Nurse Practitioner
OD	Doctor of Optometry
ONC	Orthopedic Nursing Certificate
OT	Occupational Therapist
OTL	Occupational Therapist, Licensed
OTR	Occupational Therapist, Registered
OTReg	Occupational Therapist, Registered
PA	Physician's Assistant
PBT(ASCP)	Phlebotomy Technician certified by the American Society of Clinical Pathologists
PCP	Primary Care Physician
PD	Doctor of Pharmacy
Ph.D.	Doctor of Philosophy; Doctor of Pharmacy

Chart continued on following page

PNP	Pediatric Nurse Practitioner
PT	Physical Therapist
RDA	Registered Dental Assistant
Reg	Registered
RHIA	Registered Health Information Administrator
RHIT	Registered Health Information Technician
RMA	Registered Medical Assistant
RN	Registered Nurse
RNA	Registered Nurse Anesthetist
RN, C.	Registered Nurse Certified (used to identify nurses certified by the American Nurses Credentialing Center; areas of practice are medical-surgical nurse, gerontological nurse, psychiatric and mental health nurse, pediatric nurse, perinatal nurse, community health nurse, school nurse, general nursing practice, college health nurse, gerontological nurse practitioner, pediatric nurse practitioner, adult nurse practitioner, family nurse practitioner, and school nurse practitioner)
RN, C.N.A.	Registered Nurse, Certified in Nursing Administration
RN, CNNA	Registered Nurse, Certified in Nursing Administration, Advanced
RN, C.S.	Registered Nurse, Certified Specialist (used to identify nurses certified by the American Nurses Credentialing Center; this certification recognizes clinical specialists in the following areas: gerontological nursing, medical surgical nursing, adult psychiatric and mental health nursing, child and adolescent

Professional Designations for Health Care Providers *Continued*

	psychiatric and mental health nursing, and community health nursing)
RPh	Registered Pharmacist
RPT	Registered Physical Therapist
RRL	Registered Record Librarian
RRT	Registered Respiratory Therapist
RT	Radiologic Technologist; Respiratory Therapist
RT(N)	Nuclear Medicine Technologist
RT(R)	Technologist in Diagnostic Radiology
RTR	Registered Recreational Therapist
RT(T)	Radiation Therapy Technologist
SBB(ASCP)	Specialist in Blood Banking certified by the American Society of Clinical Pathologists
ScD	Doctor of Science
SCT(ASCP)	Specialist in Cytotechnology certified by the American Society of Clinical Pathologists
SNP	School Nurse Practitioner
SW	Social Worker

The Top 100 Principal Diagnoses and Associated Principal Procedures*

Diagnosis	Most Common Associated Principal Procedures
1. Liveborn	• Circumcision • Prophylactic vaccinations and inoculations • Respiratory intubation and mechanical ventilation
2. Coronary atherosclerosis and other heart disease	• Percutaneous transluminal coronary angioplasty • Coronary artery bypass graft • Diagnostic cardiac catheterization, coronary arteriography • Cardiac stress tests
3. Pneumonia (except that caused by tuberculosis or sexually transmitted disease)	• Diagnostic bronchoscopy and biopsy of bronchus • Respiratory intubation and mechanical ventilation

* Source: Agency for Health Care Policy and Research, Center for Organization and Delivery Studies. Healthcare Cost and Utilization Project (HCUP).

Chart continued on following page

The Top 100 Principal Diagnoses and Associated Principal Procedures *Continued*

Diagnosis	Most Common Associated Principal Procedures
4. Congestive heart failure, nonhypertensive	• Diagnostic cardiac catheterization, coronary arteriography • Diagnostic ultrasound of heart (echocardiogram) • Respiratory intubation and mechanical ventilation • Incision of pleura, thoracentesis, chest drainage
5. Acute myocardial infarction	• Percutaneous transluminal coronary angioplasty • Diagnostic cardiac catheterization, coronary arteriography • Coronary artery bypass graft
6. Trauma to perineum and vulva	• Repair of current obstetrical laceration • Episiotomy • Forceps, vacuum, and breech delivery • Ligation of fallopian tubes
7. Acute cerebrovascular disease	• CT scan head • Respiratory intubation and mechanical ventilation • Gastrostomy, temporary and permanent • Magnetic resonance imaging

The Top 100 Principal Diagnoses and Associated Principal Procedures *Continued*

Diagnosis	Most Common Associated Principal Procedures
8. Normal pregnancy and/or delivery	• Episiotomy • Artificial rupture of membranes to assist delivery • Ligation of fallopian tubes
9. Affective disorders	• Psychological and psychiatric evaluation and therapy • Alcohol and drug rehabilitation/detoxification • CT scan head
10. Cardiac dysrhythmias	• Insertion, revision, replacement, removal of cardiac pace-maker or cardioverter/defibrillator • Conversion of cardiac rhythm • Diagnostic ultrasound of heart (echocardiogram)
11. Chronic obstructive pulmonary disease and bronchiectasis	• Respiratory intubation and mechanical ventilation • Diagnostic bronchoscopy and biopsy of bronchus • Arterial blood gases
12. Spondylosis, intervertebral disc disorders, other back problems	• Laminectomy, excision intervertebral disc • Spinal fusion

Chart continued on following page

Diagnosis	Most Common Associated Principal Procedures
	• Insertion of catheter or spinal stimulator and injection into spinal canal • Myelogram
13. Nonspecific chest pain	• Diagnostic cardiac catheterization, coronary arteriography • Cardiac stress tests • Diagnostic ultrasound of heart (echocardiogram) • Electrographic cardiac monitoring
14. Fluid and electrolyte disorders	• Upper gastrointestinal endoscopy, biopsy • Gastrostomy, temporary and permanent • CT scan head
15. Biliary tract disease	• Cholecystectomy and common duct exploration • Endoscopic retrograde cannulation of pancreas (ERCP)
16. Complication of device, implant or graft	• Hip replacement, total and partial • Creation, revision, and removal of arteriovenous fistula or vessel-to-vessel cannula for dialysis • Percutaneous transluminal coronary angioplasty (PTCA)

The Top 100 Principal Diagnoses and Associated Principal Procedures *Continued*

Diagnosis	Most Common Associated Principal Procedures
17. Fetal distress and abnormal forces of labor	• Cesarean section • Forceps, vacuum, and breech delivery • Episiotomy • Repair of current obstetrical laceration
18. Septicemia (except in labor)	• Diagnostic spinal tap • Blood transfusion • Debridement of wound, infection or burn
19. Asthma	• Respiratory intubation and mechanical ventilation • Arterial blood gases
20. Osteoarthritis	• Arthroplasty knee • Hip replacement, total and partial • Arthroplasty other than hip or knee
21. Urinary tract infections	• Endoscopy and endoscopic biopsy of the urinary tract • Diagnostic ultrasound of urinary tract • Diagnostic spinal tap

Chart continued on following page

The Top 100 Principal Diagnoses and Associated Principal Procedures *Continued*

Diagnosis	Most Common Associated Principal Procedures
22. Diabetes mellitus with complications	• Amputation of lower extremity • Debridement of wound, infection, or burn • Peripheral vascular bypass
23. Other complications of birth, puerperium affecting management of mother	• Episiotomy • Repair of current obstetrical laceration • Forceps, vacuum, and breech delivery • Cesarean section
24. Fracture of neck of femur	• Treatment, fracture or dislocation of hip and femur • Hip replacement, total and partial • Physical therapy exercises, manipulation, and other procedures • Traction, splints, and other wound care
25. Other complications of pregnancy	• Episiotomy • Cesarean section • Repair of current obstetrical laceration

The Top 100 Principal Diagnoses and Associated Principal Procedures *Continued*

Diagnosis	Most Common Associated Principal Procedures
26. Rehabilitation care, fitting of prostheses, and adjustment of devices	• Physical therapy exercises, manipulation, and other procedures • Diagnostic physical therapy
27. Complications of surgical procedures or medical care	• Debridement of wound, infection, or burn • Incision and drainage, skin and subcutaneous tissue • Incision of pleura, thoracentesis, chest drainage
28. Skin and subcutaneous tissue infections	• Incision and drainage, skin and subcutaneous tissue • Debridement of wound, infection, or burn
29. Gastrointestinal hemorrhage	• Upper gastrointestinal endoscopy, biopsy • Colonoscopy and biopsy • Blood transfusion
30. Alcohol-related mental disorders	• Alcohol and drug rehabilitation/detoxification • Psychological and psychiatric evaluation and therapy • CT scan head • Respiratory intubation and mechanical ventilation

Chart continued on following page

Diagnosis	Most Common Associated Principal Procedures
31. Intestinal obstruction without hernia	• Excision, lysis peritoneal adhesions • Small bowel resection • Colonoscopy and biopsy • Nasogastric tube
32. Fracture of lower limb	• Treatment, fracture or dislocation of lower extremity (other than hip or femur) • Treatment, fracture or dislocation of hip and femur • Traction, splints, and other wound care • Debridement of wound, infection, or burn
33. Early or threatened labor	• Cesarean section • Episiotomy • Fetal monitoring
34. Previous cesarean section	• Cesarean section • Episiotomy

The Top 100 Principal Diagnoses and Associated Principal Procedures *Continued*

Diagnosis	Most Common Associated Principal Procedures
35. Umbilical cord complication	• Forceps, vacuum, and breech delivery • Repair of current obstetrical laceration • Episiotomy • Repair of current obstetrical laceration • Forceps, vacuum, and breech delivery • Artificial rupture of membranes to assist delivery
36. Secondary malignancies	• Incision of pleura, thoracentesis, chest drainage • Therapeutic radiology • Cancer chemotherapy
37. Maintenance chemotherapy, radiotherapy	• Cancer chemotherapy • Therapeutic radiology
38. Schizophrenia and related disorders	• Psychological and psychiatric evaluation and therapy • Alcohol and drug rehabilitation/detoxification • CT scan head

Chart continued on following page

The Top 100 Principal Diagnoses and Associated Principal Procedures *Continued*

Diagnosis	Most Common Associated Principal Procedures
39. Hypertension with complications and secondary hypertension	• Hemodialysis • Creation, revision and removal of arteriovenous fistula or vessel-to-vessel cannula for dialysis • Diagnostic cardiac catheterization, coronary arteriography • Diagnostic ultrasound of heart (echocardiogram)
40. Substance-related mental disorders	• Alcohol and drug rehabilitation/detoxification • Psychological and psychiatric evaluation and therapy • CT scan head • Diagnostic spinal tap
41. Diverticulosis and diverticulitis	• Colorectal resection • Colonoscopy and biopsy • Upper gastrointestinal endoscopy, biopsy • CT scan abdomen
42. Benign neoplasm of uterus	• Hysterectomy, abdominal and vaginal • Diagnostic dilatation and curettage • Oophorectomy, unilateral and bilateral

The Top 100 Principal Diagnoses and Associated Principal Procedures *Continued*

Diagnosis	Most Common Associated Principal Procedures
43. Appendicitis and other appendiceal conditions	• Appendectomy • Colorectal resection • Excision, lysis peritoneal adhesions
44. Epilepsy, convulsions	• CT scan head • Respiratory intubation and mechanical ventilation • Diagnostic spinal tap • Electroencephalogram (EEG)
45. Polyhydramnios and other problems of amniotic cavity	• Episiotomy • Cesarean section • Repair of current obstetrical laceration • Forceps, vacuum, and breech delivery
46. Acute bronchitis	• Diagnostic spinal tap • Diagnostic bronchoscopy and biopsy of bronchus
47. Respiratory failure, insufficiency, arrest	• Respiratory intubation and mechanical ventilation

Chart continued on following page

The Top 100 Principal Diagnoses and Associated Principal Procedures *Continued*

Diagnosis	Most Common Associated Principal Procedures
	• Tracheostomy, temporary and permanent • Diagnostic bronchoscopy and biopsy of bronchus
48. Pancreatic disorders (not diabetes)	• Cholecystectomy and common duct exploration • Upper gastrointestinal endoscopy, biopsy • Endoscopic retrograde cannulation of pancreas (ERCP)
49. Transient cerebral ischemia	• CT scan head • Diagnostic ultrasound of heart (echocardiogram) • Diagnostic ultrasound of head and neck • Magnetic resonance imaging
50. Syncope	• CT scan head • Diagnostic ultrasound of heart (echocardiogram)
51. Phlebitis, thrombophlebitis and thromboembolism	• Arteriogram or venogram (not heart and head)
52. Calculus of urinary tract	• Transurethral excision, drainage, or removal urinary obstruction

The Top 100 Principal Diagnoses and Associated Principal Procedures *Continued*

Diagnosis	Most Common Associated Principal Procedures
	• Ureteral catheterization • Intravenous pyelogram • Endoscopy and endoscopic biopsy of the urinary tract
53. Hypertension complicating pregnancy, childbirth and the puerperium	• Cesarean section • Episiotomy • Forceps, vacuum, and breech delivery
54. Aspiration pneumonitis, food/vomitus	• Respiratory intubation and mechanical ventilation • Gastrostomy, temporary and permanent • Upper gastrointestinal endoscopy, biopsy • Diagnostic bronchoscopy and biopsy of bronchus
55. Occlusion or stenosis of precerebral arteries	• Endarterectomy, vessel of head and neck • Cerebral arteriogram • CT scan head
56. Intracranial injury	• CT scan head • Suture of skin and subcutaneous tissue

Chart continued on following page

The Top 100 Principal Diagnoses and Associated Principal Procedures *Continued*

Diagnosis	Most Common Associated Principal Procedures
57. Other fractures	• Incision and excision of central nervous system (CNS) • Respiratory intubation and mechanical ventilation
58. Other lower respiratory disease	• Suture of skin and subcutaneous tissue • Physical therapy exercises, manipulation, and other procedures • Diagnostic bronchoscopy and biopsy of bronchus • Diagnostic cardiac catheterization, coronary arteriography • Lobectomy or pneumonectomy
59. Abdominal hernia	• Inguinal and femoral hernia repair • Excision, lysis peritoneal adhesions
60. Cancer of bronchus, lung	• Lobectomy or pneumonectomy • Diagnostic bronchoscopy and biopsy of bronchus • Incision of pleura, thoracentesis, chest drainage • Therapeutic radiology
61. Esophageal disorders	• Upper gastrointestinal endoscopy, biopsy

The Top 100 Principal Diagnoses and Associated Principal Procedures *Continued*

Diagnosis	Most Common Associated Principal Procedures
	• Diagnostic cardiac catheterization, coronary arteriography
	• Esophageal dilatation
62. Prolapse of female genital organs	• Hysterectomy, abdominal and vaginal
	• Repair of cystocele and rectocele, obliteration of vaginal vault
	• Genitourinary incontinence procedures
	• Oophorectomy, unilateral and bilateral
63. Malposition, malpresentation	• Cesarean section
	• Forceps, vacuum, and breech delivery
	• Episiotomy
	• Repair of current obstetrical laceration
64. Other gastrointestinal disorders	• Colonoscopy and biopsy
	• Colorectal resection
	• Upper gastrointestinal endoscopy, biopsy
65. Abdominal pain	• Upper gastrointestinal endoscopy, biopsy
	• Appendectomy

Chart continued on following page

Diagnosis	Most Common Associated Principal Procedures
	• CT scan abdomen • Colonoscopy and biopsy
66. Other and unspecified benign neoplasm	• Oophorectomy, unilateral and bilateral • Hysterectomy, abdominal and vaginal • Thyroidectomy, partial or complete • Colorectal resection
67. Fetopelvic disproportion, obstruction	• Cesarean section • Forceps, vacuum, and breech delivery • Episiotomy • Repair of current obstetrical laceration
68. Other mental conditions	• Psychological and psychiatric evaluation and therapy • Alcohol and drug rehabilitation/detoxification • Suture of skin and subcutaneous tissue
69. Gastritis and duodenitis	• Upper gastrointestinal endoscopy, biopsy • Colonoscopy and biopsy • Blood transfusion

The Top 100 Principal Diagnoses and Associated Principal Procedures *Continued*

Diagnosis	Most Common Associated Principal Procedures
70. Fracture of upper limb	• Treatment, fracture or dislocation of radius and ulna • Arthroplasty other than hip or knee • Traction, splints, and other wound care
71. Peripheral and visceral atherosclerosis	• Peripheral vascular bypass • Colonoscopy and biopsy • Colorectal resection
72. Senility and organic mental disorders	• CT scan head • Psychological and psychiatric evaluation and therapy • Diagnostic spinal tap • Magnetic resonance imaging
73. Noninfectious gastroenteritis	• Colonoscopy and biopsy • Upper gastrointestinal endoscopy, biopsy • CT scan abdomen
74. HIV infection	• Diagnostic bronchoscopy and biopsy of bronchus • Diagnostic spinal tap • Blood transfusion

Chart continued on following page

The Top 100 Principal Diagnoses and Associated Principal Procedures *Continued*

Diagnosis	Most Common Associated Principal Procedures
75. Cancer of breast	• Mastectomy • Lumpectomy, quadrantectomy of breast • Breast biopsy and other diagnostic procedures on breast
76. Poisoning by other medications and drugs	• Respiratory intubation and mechanical ventilation • Electrographic cardiac monitoring • CT scan head
77. Intestinal infection	• Colonoscopy and biopsy • Upper gastrointestinal endoscopy, biopsy • Diagnostic spinal tap
78. Hyperplasia of prostate	• Transurethral resection of prostate • Open prostatectomy • Endoscopy and endoscopic biopsy of the urinary tract • Procedures on the urethra
79. Cancer of colon	• Colorectal resection • Colonoscopy and biopsy • Upper gastrointestinal endoscopy, biopsy

The Top 100 Principal Diagnoses and Associated Principal Procedures *Continued*

Diagnosis	Most Common Associated Principal Procedures
80. Other female genital disorders	• Hysterectomy, abdominal and vaginal • Genitourinary incontinence procedures • Oophorectomy, unilateral and bilateral
81. Cancer of prostate	• Open prostatectomy • Transurethral resection of prostate
82. Other nervous system disorders	• Diagnostic spinal tap • CT scan head • Magnetic resonance imaging
83. Forceps delivery	• Forceps, vacuum, and breech delivery • Repair of current obstetrical laceration • Episiotomy
84. Other connective tissue disease	• Arthroplasty other than hip or knee • Debridement of wound, infection or burn

Chart continued on following page

Diagnosis	Most Common Associated Principal Procedures
85. Pleurisy, pneumothorax, pulmonary collapse	• Incision of pleura, thoracentesis, chest drainage • Lobectomy or pneumonectomy • Diagnostic bronchoscopy and biopsy of bronchus
86. Viral infection	• Diagnostic spinal tap • Upper gastrointestinal endoscopy, biopsy • CT scan head
87. Prolonged pregnancy	• Episiotomy • Cesarean section • Forceps, vacuum, and breech delivery • Repair of current obstetrical laceration
88. Deficiency and other anemia	• Blood transfusion • Upper gastrointestinal endoscopy, biopsy • Bone marrow biopsy • Colonoscopy and biopsy
89. Crushing injury or internal injury	• Incision of pleura, thoracentesis, chest drainage

The Top 100 Principal Diagnoses and Associated Principal Procedures *Continued*

Diagnosis	Most Common Associated Principal Procedures
90. Heart valve disorders	• Heart valve procedures • Diagnostic cardiac catheterization, coronary arteriography • Diagnostic ultrasound of heart (echocardiogram)
91. Other circulatory disease	• Peripheral vascular bypass • Diagnostic cardiac catheterization, coronary arteriography
92. Acute and unspecified renal failure	• Hemodialysis • Creation, revision and removal of arterioverous fistula or vessel-to-vessel cannula for dialysis • Upper gastrointestinal endoscopy, biopsy
93. Endometriosis	• Hysterectomy, abdominal and vaginal • Oophorectomy, unilateral and bilateral
94. Other bone disease and musculoskeletal deformities	• Hip replacement, total and partial • Spinal fusion • Partial excision bone

Chart continued on following page

The Top 100 Principal Diagnoses and Associated Principal Procedures *Continued*

Diagnosis	Most Common Associated Principal Procedures
95. Sprains and strains	• Arthroplasty knee • Arthroplasty other than hip or knee
96. Other upper respiratory infections	• Diagnostic spinal tap
97. Pulmonary heart disease	• Radioisotope pulmonary scan • Arteriogram or venogram (not heart and head) • Diagnostic cardiac catheterization, coronary arteriography
98. Pericarditis, endocarditis, and myo-carditis, cardiomyopathy (except that caused by tuberculosis or sexually transmitted disease)	• Diagnostic cardiac catheterization, coronary arteriography • Diagnostic ultrasound of heart (echocardiogram)
99. Aortic, peripheral, and visceral artery aneurysms	• Aortic resection, replacement or anastomosis • Peripheral vascular bypass
100. Other injuries and conditions due to external causes	• Upper gastrointestinal endoscopy, biopsy • CT scan head • Nonoperative removal of foreign body • Respiratory intubation and mechanical ventilation

The Top 100 Prescription Drugs (Listed Alphabetically)*[1]

Trade Name[2]	Generic Name	Type/Use	Rank[3]
Accupril	quinapril	Antihypertensive (ACE inhibitor)	41
Acetaminophen/Codeine (Tylenol with Codeine)	acetaminophen/codeine	Nonnarcotic analgesic; antipyretic	24 (Teva Pharm) 95 (Purepac)
Adalat CC	nifedipine	Calcium channel blocker (antianginal and antihypertensive)	77

* Adapted from American Druggist, February 1999, pp 42–43.
[1] Based on more than 2.4 billion U.S. prescriptions in 1998.
[2] Names in parentheses in this column are the most recognizable trade names for drugs that are available generically.
[3] Names in parentheses in this column are the different manufacturers of the same drug, each next to their respective ranking within the top 100.

Chart continued on following page

The Top 100 Prescription Drugs (Listed Alphabetically) Continued

Trade Name[2]	Generic Name	Type/Use	Rank[3]
Albuterol Aerosol	albuterol	Bronchodilator	13
Albuterol Neb Soln	albuterol	Bronchodilator	82
Allegra	fexofenadine	Antihistamine	56
Alprazolam (Xanax)	alprazolam	Antianxiety (benzodiazepine tranquilizer)	38 (Greenstone) 73 (Geneva)
Ambien	zolpidem	Sedative-hypnotic (for insomnia)	39
Amitriptyline (Elavil)	amitriptyline	Antidepressant (tricyclic)	66
Amoxicillin	amoxicillin	Antibiotic (penicillin-type)	15
Amoxil	amoxicillin	Antibiotic (penicillin-type)	40
Atenolol (Tenormin)	atenolol	Beta-blocker (antihypertensive and antiarrhythmic)	62 (Geneva) 75 (Mylan) 79 (ESI Lederle)

The Top 100 Prescription Drugs (Listed Alphabetically) Continued

Trade Name[2]	Generic Name	Type/Use	Rank[3]
Atrovent	ipratropium	Bronchodilator	97
Augmentin	amoxicillin/clavulanate	Antibiotic (penicillin-type)	19
Biaxin	clarithromycin	Antibiotic (erythromycin-type)	31
Cardizem CD	diltiazem	Calcium channel blocker	29
Cardura	doxazosin	Antihypertensive	54
Carisoprodol (Soma)	carisoprodol	Skeletal muscle relaxant	89
Ceftin	cefuroxime	Antibiotic (cephalosporin-type)	92
Cefzil	cefprozil	Antibiotic (cephalosporin-type)	67
Cephalexin (Keflex)	cephalexin	Antibiotic (cephalosporin-type)	20

Chart continued on following page

169

The Top 100 Prescription Drugs (Listed Alphabetically) Continued

Trade Name[2]	Generic Name	Type/Use	Rank[3]
Cipro	ciprofloxacin	Anti-infective (quinolone-type)	27
Claritin	loratadine	Antihistamine and decongestant	10
Claritin-D 12 HR	loratadine/pseudoephedrine	Antihistamine and decongestant	55
Claritin-D 24 HR	loratadine/pseudoephedrine	Antihistamine and decongestant	93
Clonazepam (Klonopin)	clonazepam	Anticonvulsant (benzodiazepine)	87
Coumadin	warfarin	Anticoagulant	23
Cozaar	losartan	Antihypertensive (Angiotensin II receptor antagonist)	78

The Top 100 Prescription Drugs (Listed Alphabetically) *Continued*

Trade Name[2]	Generic Name	Type/Use	Rank[3]
Daypro	oxaprozin	Nonsteroidal anti-inflammatory drug (NSAID) (for rheumatoid arthritis and osteoarthritis)	90
Depakote	divalproex	Anticonvulsant and antimanic	68
Diflucan	fluconazole	Antifungal	71
Dilantin	phenytoin	Anticonvulsant	60
Flonase	fluticasone	Corticosteroid	64
Fosamax	alendronate	Bone resorption inhibitor; calcium regulator	76
Furosemide (Lasix)	furosemide	Diuretic (CHF and fluid accumulation)	26

Chart continued on following page

The Top 100 Prescription Drugs (Listed Alphabetically) *Continued*

Trade Name[2]	Generic Name	Type/Use	Rank[3]
Glucophage	metformin	Antidiabetic (biguanide antihyperglycemic)	22
Glucotrol XL	glipizide	Oral sulfonylurea (antidiabetic)	43
Glyburide (Micronase)	glyburide	Antidiabetic (oral hypoglycemic)	83
Humulin 70/30	human insulin 70/30	Antidiabetic (hypoglycemic: Types 1 and 2 diabetes)	98
Humulin N	human insulin-NPH	Antidiabetic (hypoglycemic)	59
Hydrochlorothiazide (HydroDIURIL)	hydrochlorothiazide	Diuretic (for CHF and hypertension)	94
Hydrocodone w/APAP (Percocet, Percodan)	hydrocodone w/APAP	Narcotic analgesic (opioid)	4 (Watson) 44 (Mallinckrodt) 81 (Qualitest)

The Top 100 Prescription Drugs (Listed Alphabetically) Continued

Trade Name[2]	Generic Name	Type/Use	Rank[3]
Hytrin	terazosin	Antihypertensive and for BPH (relaxes bladder muscle)	49
Ibuprofen	ibuprofen	Nonsteroidal anti-inflammatory drug (NSAID)	25
Imdur	isosorbide mononitrate	Nitrate (for angina pectoris)	69
K-Dur 20	potassium chloride	Electrolyte	42
Lanoxin	digoxin	Cardiotonic and antiarrhythmic	11
Lescol	fluvastatin	Cholesterol lowering agent	80
Levoxyl	levothyroxine	Thyroid hormone	33
Lipitor	atorvastatin	Cholesterol lowering agent	8

Chart continued on following page

The Top 100 Prescription Drugs (Listed Alphabetically) Continued

Trade Name[2]	Generic Name	Type/Use	Rank[3]
Lorazepam (Ativan)	lorazepam	Antianxiety (benzodiazepine tranquilizer)	65
Lotensin	benazepril	Antihypertensive (ACE inhibitor)	47
Lotrisone	clotrimazole/betamethasone	Antifungal	100
Monopril	fosinopril	Antihypertensive (ACE inhibitor)	91
Naproxen	naproxen	Nonsteroidal anti-inflammatory drug (NSAID)	88
Nitrostat	nitroglycerin	Nitrate (anti-anginal)	96
Norvasc	amlodipine	Antihypertensive (calcium channel blocker)	9

The Top 100 Prescription Drugs (Listed Alphabetically) *Continued*

Trade Name[2]	Generic Name	Type/Use	Rank[3]
Ortho-Novum 7/7/7	low-dose estrogen/low-dose progestin	Contraceptive	61
Ortho Tri-Cyclen	low-dose estrogen/low-dose progestin	Pregnancy prevention (contraceptive)	46
Paxil	paroxetine	Antidepressant (SSRI)	14
Pepcid	famotidine	H-2 receptor antagonist	57
Pravachol	pravastatin	Cholesterol lowering agent	30
Prednisone	prednisone	Corticosteroid	35
Premarin	estrogen	Hormone (female)	1
Prempro	conjugated estrogen/medroxyprogesterone	Hormone (female) (HRT)	16

Chart continued on following page

The Top 100 Prescription Drugs (Listed Alphabetically) Continued

Trade Name[2]	Generic Name	Type/Use	Rank[3]
Prevacid	lansoprazole	Gastric acid pump inhibitor	36
Prilosec	omeprazole	Gastric acid pump inhibitor	6
Prinivil	lisinopril	Antihypertensive (ACE inhibitor)	48
Procardia XL	nifedipine	Calcium channel blocker	34
Propoxyphene N/APAP (Darvon, Darvocet)	propoxyphene N/APAP	Narcotic analgesic (opioid)	32 (Mylan) 51 (Teva Pharm)
Propulsid	cisapride	Gastrointestinal stimulant (for GERD)	72
Prozac	fluoxetine	Antidepressant (SSRI)	5
Relafen	nabumetone	Nonsteroidal anti-inflammatory drug (NSAID)	52

The Top 100 Prescription Drugs (Listed Alphabetically) *Continued*

Trade Name[2]	Generic Name	Type/Use	Rank[3]
Rezulin	troglitazone	Antidiabetic (hypoglycemic: Type 2 diabetes)	99
Synthroid	levothyroxine	Thyroid hormone	2
Toprol-XL	metoprolol	Antihypertensive (beta-blocker)	63
Triamterene/HCTZ (Dyazide)	triamterene/HCTZ	Diuretic (Potassium sparing)	45 (Geneva) 74 (Mylan)
Trimethoprim/Sulfa (Septra, Bactrim)	trimethoprim/sulfameth-oxazole	Anti-infective	28
Trimox	amoxicillin	Antibiotic (penicillin-type)	3
Triphasil	low-dose estrogen/low-dose progestin	Contraceptive	58

Chart continued on following page

The Top 100 Prescription Drugs (Listed Alphabetically) *Continued*

Trade Name[2]	Generic Name	Type/Use	Rank[3]
Ultram	tramadol	Non-narcotic analgesic	37
Vancenase AQ DS	beclomethasone	Corticosteroid and anti-inflammatory (nasal spray)	85
Vasotec	enalapril	Antihypertensive (ACE inhibitor)	18
Veetids	penicillin VK	Antibiotic (penicillin-type)	50
Viagra	sildenafil citrate	Vasodilator (for erectile dysfunction)	70
Wellbutrin SR	bupropion	Antidepressant; smoking cessation aid	84
Zestril	lisinopril	Antihypertensive (ACE inhibitor)	17
Zithromax	azithromycin	Antibiotic (erythromycin-type)	7

The Top 100 Prescription Drugs (Listed Alphabetically) *Continued*

Trade Name[2]	Generic Name	Type/Use	Rank[3]
Zithromax Susp	azithromycin	Antibiotic (erythromycin-type)	86
Zocor	simvastatin	Cholesterol lowering agent	21
Zoloft	sertraline	Antidepressant (SSRI)	12
Zyrtec	cetirizine	Antihistamine	53

Abbreviations:

ACE = angiotensin-converting enzyme
APAP = acetaminophen
BPH = benign prostatic hyperplasia

CHF = congestive heart failure
GERD = gastroesophageal reflux disease
HCTZ = hydrochlorothiazide

N = napsylate
NPH = isophane insulin
SSRI = selective serotonin receptor inhibitor

Normal Hematological Reference Values and Implications of Abnormal Results*

The implications of abnormal results are major ones in each category. SI units are the International System of Units that are generally accepted for all scientific and technical uses.

cu mm = cubic millimeter (mm^3)
dL = deciliter (1/10 liter or 100 mL)
g = gram
L = liter
mg = milligram (1/1000 gram)
mL = milliliter
mEq = milliequivalent
mill = million
mm = millimeter (1/1000 meter)
mmol = millimole
thou = thousand
U = unit
μmol = micromole (one-millionth of a mole)

---

*From Chabner DE: The Language of Medicine, 6th ed. Philadelphia, W.B. Saunders, 2001.

Cell Counts*

	Conventional Units	SI Units	Implications
Erythrocytes (RBC)			*High* • Polycythemia
Females	4.2–5.4 million/mm^3	4.2–5.4 × 10^{12}/L	• Dehydration
Males	4.6–6.2 million/mm^3	4.6–6.2 × 10^{12}/L	*Low* • Iron deficiency anemia
Children	4.5–5.1 million/mm^3	4.5–5.1 × 10^{12}/L	• Blood loss
Leukocytes (WBC)			*High* • Bacterial infection
Total	4500–11,000/mm^3	4.5–11.0 × 10^9/L	• Leukemia
			• Eosinophils high in allergy
Differential	%		*Low* • Viral infection
Neutrophils	54–62		• Aplastic anemia
Lymphocytes	20–40		• Chemotherapy
Monocytes	3–7		
Eosinophils	1–3		
Basophils	0–1		

*From Chabner DE: The Language of Medicine, 6th ed. Philadelphia, W.B. Saunders, 2001.

Chart continued on following page

Cell Counts *Continued*

	Conventional Units	SI Units	Implications
Platelets	200,000–400,000/mm³	200–400 × 10⁹/L	*High* • Hemorrhage • Infections • Malignancy • Splenectomy *Low* • Aplastic anemia • Chemotherapy • Hypersplenism

Coagulation Tests*

	Conventional Units	SI Units	Implications
Bleeding Time (template method)	2.75–8.0 min	2.75–8.0 min	*Prolonged* • Aspirin ingestion • Low platelet count
Coagulation Time	5–15 min	5–15 min	*Prolonged* • Heparin therapy
Prothrombin Time (PT)	12–14 sec	12–14 sec	*Prolonged* • Vitamin K deficiency • Hepatic disease • Oral anticoagulant therapy

* From Chabner DE: The Language of Medicine, 6th ed. Philadelphia, W.B. Saunders, 2001.

Red Blood Cell Tests*

	Conventional Units	SI Units	Implications
Hematocrit (Hct)			
Females	37–47%	0.37–0.47	*High* • Polycythemia
Males	40–54%	0.40–0.54	• Dehydration
			Low • Loss of blood
			• Anemia
Hemoglobin (Hgb)			
Females	12.0–14.0 gm/dL	1.86–2.48 mmol/L	*High* • Polycythemia
Males	14.0–16.0 gm/dL	2.17–2.79 mmol/L	• Dehydration
			Low • Anemia
			• Blood loss

* From Chabner DE: The Language of Medicine, 6th ed. Philadelphia, W.B. Saunders, 2001.

Serum Tests*

	Conventional Units	SI Units	Implications	
Alanine aminotransferase (ALT, SGPT)	5–30 U/L	5–30 U/L	*High*	• Hepatitis
Albumin	3.5–5.5 gm/dL	35–55 g/L	*Low*	• Hepatic disease • Malnutrition • Nephritis and nephrosis
Alkaline phosphatase (ALP)	20–90 U/L	20–90 U/L	*High*	• Bone disease • Hepatitis or tumor infiltration of liver • Biliary obstruction
Aspartate aminotransferase (AST, SGOT)	10–30 U/L	10–30 U/L	*High*	• Hepatitis • Cardiac and muscle injury

---

*From Chabner DE: The Language of Medicine, 6th ed. Philadelphia, W.B. Saunders, 2001.

Chart continued on following page

Serum Tests *Continued*

	Conventional Units	SI Units	Implications
Bilirubin			
Total	0.3–1.1 mg/dL	5.1–19 μmol/L	*High* • Hemolysis
Neonates	1–12 mg/dL	17–205 μmol/L	• Neonatal hepatic immaturity
			• Cirrhosis
			• Biliary tract obstruction
Blood urea nitrogen (BUN)	8–20 mg/dL	3.0–7.1 mmol/L	*High* • Renal disease
			• Reduced renal blood flow
			• Urinary tract obstruction
			Low • Hepatic damage
			• Malnutrition
Calcium	9.0–11.0 mg/dL	2.23–2.75 mmol/L	*High* • Hyperparathyroidism
			• Multiple myeloma
			• Metastatic cancer
			Low • Hypoparathyroidism
			• Total parathyroidectomy

Serum Tests *Continued*

	Conventional Units	SI Units	Implications
Cholesterol			*High* • High fat diet
Desirable range	<200 mg/dL	<5.18 mmol/L	• Inherited
LDL cholesterol	60–80 mg/dL	600–1800 mg/L	hypercholesterolemia
HDL cholesterol	30–80 mg/dL	300–800 mg/L	*Low* • Starvation
Creatine phosphokinase (CPK)			*High* • Myocardial infarction
Females	30–135 U/L	30–135 U/L	• Musc.e disease
Males	55–170 U/L	55–170 U/L	*High* • Renal disease
Creatinine	0.6–1.2 mg/dL	53–106 µmol/L	*High* • Diabetes mellitus
Glucose (fasting)	70–115 mg/dL	3.89–6.38 mmol/L	*High* • Hyperinsulinism
			Low • Fasting
			• Hypothyroidism
			• Addison disease
			• Pituitary insufficiency

Chart continued on following page

Serum Tests *Continued*

	Conventional Units	SI Units	Implications
Lactate dehydrogenase (LDH)	100–190 U/L	100–190 U/L	*High* • Tissue necrosis • Myocardial infarction • Liver disease • Muscle disease
Phosphate ($-PO_4$)	3.0–4.5 mg/dL	1.0–1.5 mmol/L	*High* • Renal failure • Bone metastases • Hypoparathyroidism *Low* • Malnutrition • Malabsorption • Hyperparathyroidism
Potassium (K)	3.5–5.0 mEq/L	3.5–5.0 mmol/L	*High* • Burn victims • Renal failure • Diabetic ketoacidosis *Low* • Cushing syndrome • Loss of body fluids

Serum Tests *Continued*

	Conventional Units	SI Units	Implications
Sodium (Na)	136–145 mEq/L	136–145 mmol/L	*High* • Inadequate water intake • Water loss in excess of sodium *Low* • Adrenal insufficiency • Inadequate sodium intake • Excessive sodium loss
Thyroxine (T₄)	4.4–9.9 μg/dL	57–128 nmol/L	*High* • Graves disease (hyperthyroidism) *Low* • Hypothyroidism
Uric acid Females Males	1.5–7.0 mg/dL 2.5–8.0 mg/dL	0.09–0.42 mmol/L 0.15–0.48 mmol/L	*High* • Gout • Leukemia

PART III

BODY SYSTEMS ILLUSTRATIONS*

* Illustrations adapted from Chabner DE: The Language of Medicine, 6th ed. Philadelphia, W.B. Saunders, 2001.

Index of Body Systems Illustrations

This is an index of all the important labels in the following illustrations of the body systems. You can use it to locate the relevant illustration for a particular anatomical term you may have in mind.

THE CARDIOVASCULAR SYSTEM (AORTA AND MAJOR ARTERIES)

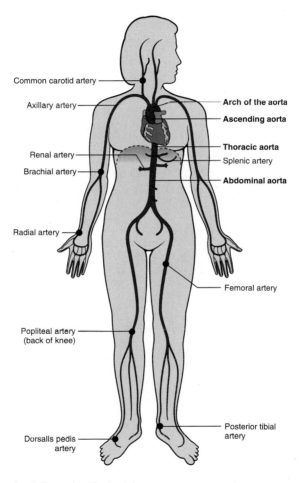

Common carotid artery

Axillary artery

Arch of the aorta

Ascending aorta

Thoracic aorta

Renal artery

Splenic artery

Brachial artery

Abdominal aorta

Radial artery

Femoral artery

Popliteal artery
(back of knee)

Posterior tibial
artery

Dorsalls pedis
artery

Dots indicate pulse points in arteries

THE CARDIOVASCULAR SYSTEM (HEART)

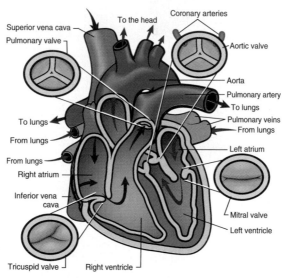

Superior vena cava

Pulmonary valve

To the head

Coronary arteries

Aortic valve

Aorta

Pulmonary artery

To lungs

Pulmonary veins

From lungs

To lungs

From lungs

From lungs

Left atrium

Right atrium

Inferior vena cava

Mitral valve

Left ventricle

Tricuspid valve

Right ventricle

RIGHT SIDE OF THE HEART   LEFT SIDE OF THE HEART